From Outside the Closet

Stories of Men Who Love Men

*Always strive to be
your true self!*

A.C. xx

Anne Considine

Cover design: Ultimate World Publishing
Layout and typesetting: Ultimate World Publishing
Editor: Isabelle Russell

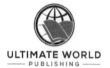

Ultimate World Publishing
Diamond Creek,
Victoria Australia 3089
www.writeabook.com.au

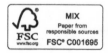

The paper in this book is FSC® certified. FSC® promotes environmentally responsible, socially beneficial and economically viable management of the world's forests.

MIX
Paper from responsible sources
FSC® C001695

Testimonials

"A collection of brave stories beautifully presented with both raw honesty and sensitivity. Insightful and thought provoking – a wonderful read encouraging greater acceptance, compassion and understanding."

Sue Dyson

"Engaging portraits of several men who on their journeys through childhood to adulthood where they feel out of sync with mainstream culture. Heartbreaking, heartwarming and insightful stories about growing up gay in Australia. Anne has presented the opportunity for greater understanding and acceptance of this faction of society with tact and sensitivity, and we should look forward to more of her work in the future."

Margaret Burn

Dedication

To the beautiful men who found the courage to be their true selves and live their lives with purpose, meaning and integrity.

Contents

Introduction

I believe there is a reason we were all put on this earth: to make a difference to people's lives, hopefully for the better. Some are destined to be famous, some infamous, but most of us are here to influence those around us – and that's enough too. If you can brighten up someone's life, or even just their day, then that is as good an act as you can do for humanity. However, when we get caught up in the everyday hustle and bustle of life, we sometimes forget to treat our family and friends with the love and care they deserve. On top of this, there are the negative influences from family, friends and society who believe they know what's best for everyone else and how they should behave.

This brings me to why I decided to write this book. Having our two sons come out as gay turned my husband's and my world on its axis for a short time as we came to terms with the change in our family dynamic. Please don't get me wrong, this was not about whether we accepted them or not. Rather, it was about us reconceptualising the traditional family we thought we had and where it was heading, how that had been changed somewhat and its direction altered. Not a wrong direction, just a different direction. Instead of potentially having two daughters-in-law and one son-in-law, we now hope to have three sons-in-law! That was 14 years ago.

When our first son came out, I wanted to find out more about the gay community and lifestyle as we had not previously been immersed in the culture. Back then there was not as much information or books as there is now, and what I did find didn't make me feel any more confident of the future health and wellbeing of my two boys. It was quite a seedy experience Googling 'gay' for information back in the early 2000s. So, I wanted to create a book that tells stories of gay men who have come out, and what they have learnt about themselves, and any helpful information or insights they can pass on to help others who may be currently struggling with their sexuality. I have included a couple of stories of parents' experiences which may help other parents who have felt a bit out of their depth and unsure of how to move forward.

I've had many people over the years tell me that if their child was gay it would be, 'No big deal, not a problem at all.' Well, what I want to say is that until that person is standing in my shoes, then they have no idea how they will react. I will always love my boys no matter what and have their best interests at heart, but as a mother, all I could think about at first was about their mental health, that they could face discrimination, their risk of contracting HIV, the party, alcohol and drug scene and the difficulty of finding a partner in a diminished dating pool compared to the options heterosexuals have – let alone my coming to terms with the fact that I always thought I'd be surrounded by lots of grandchildren. I know that can still be on the cards, but the reality is that there is a much lower chance of this happening now; selfish maybe, but true for me nonetheless. So, I suggest that you don't ever assume how you will react and tell someone in that situation that's it's not a big deal!

Intrinsically, humans want to be accepted and loved for who they are. Yet, even in today's society, this is not always the case in relation to the LGBTIQ (lesbian, gay, bisexual, transgender, intersex and queer) community. A classic example is the AFL (Australian Football League) as not one player to date has come out while playing, yet the statistics indicate that 1 in 10 people is gay. Quite frankly, I don't blame someone for not coming out in the AFL, as I'm sure they'd be targeted by the opposing fans with foul comments spraying out of their mouths. The suicide rate is three to six times higher in the younger LGBTIQ demographic compared to suicides in the younger general population. What the hell is going on, people! There is no quick fix for this issue, but we can all be kinder and more accepting of each other's differences no matter what they may be, making the world a better, more tolerant place to live.

I can imagine that coming out would be one of the hardest things to do in this world that straight people will never have to experience. This is why I love it when I see gay men living happy and authentic lives because they can just be themselves – nothing to prove to anyone! I would like to encourage everyone in the gay community to be true to themselves. I take my hat off to you all as you are very brave souls, even in this day and age.

What I would like you to do is sit back and embrace the stories of these amazing men who have risen above the challenges in their life and want to inspire others to do the same!

Lindsay

The younger years

I grew up in Warracknabeal, a small Victorian town located about four hours from Melbourne towards the South Australian border. I have a sister, Sarah, who is seven years younger than me. My parents split up when I was 15 years old.

Dad worked for Australia Post his whole life and Mum is an accountant. She grew her own accounting business from when I was about two years old. Five years later when Sarah was born, Dad retired to stay home and look after us kids as Mum's accounting business was going well. Around the age of 12, it was becoming obvious that Dad had emotionally checked out from the family. Mum had tried everything to get him to engage, but to no avail. We started going on family holidays without him. He neglected to watch us play community sport and his moods were becoming detached from empathy and love. Looking back, I can see now that my father has struggled with what I would call depressive symptoms for most of my life. He's not able to cope with his feelings, so back then he just shut himself off from the family. This had a major effect on me and as he got grumpier and grumpier; we regularly butted heads. I was never good enough for him and could never be the son he wanted me to be. He wanted a tough son who loved football, lived a traditional life by getting married and having children to pass on the family name to, who would in turn give him grandchildren, and continue to live in the country. This pressure was, and has been, crippling for me, and a big reason I had no intention of ever 'coming out'. This life that he wanted for me was not how I saw my life playing out, but I desperately wanted to be accepted by him. To try and fit in with his expectations, I even had posters of half-naked women all over the walls in my room at home to pretend as though I was a rough hetero man, rather than a sensitive gay teen. Some things you just can't fake though, and this 'straight' acting was exhausting. High school was a difficult time as I became a teenager and started to experiment with who I was. Kids can be cruel and anyone that is different in the country quickly has it pointed out to them.

By the age of 15, I decided I wanted to go to boarding school for a fresh start. This was my way of moving away from the bullying and teasing from kids at school about me being gay. I never told my parents about the incidents at school (specifically the gay bullying) and persuaded them that it was to improve my education. As I was fairly academic, I don't think they thought it was for any other reason, and so I was enrolled at one of the closest boarding schools to home, over 250 km away.

I was housed in a dormitory with five other boys and unbeknownst to me, one of them, Dave, was openly gay – at 15! What courage. How ironic, though, that this was the boy that I

6

instantly connected with; he was so lovely and invited to show me around the school and local area (at this point I didn't know he was gay). This instant connection though tarnished me with the gay brush within two days of my arrival at my new school. What the hell was the universe doing to me? I remember one of the first days of school, Dave and I walked down to the local shops as you do as a teenager with no money. Then, later that evening as I sat down in the massive dining hall for dinner, some of the other boys started asking me if I was gay. What the fuck! How did they know? I denied it at all costs. They went on to explain to me that Dave was gay, and that they thought I was too because we had been hanging out. From then on, I avoided Dave like the plague to take the heat off myself. Even though I knew it to be true, I was deep in the closet and the thought of coming out was not even in my peripheral. At this point in my school life, I was an overachiever and my grades reflected my hard work and dedication. As the months progressed into my time at boarding school though, this started to change as all my effort went into fitting in with the straight boys. I tried playing footy again, began partying on weekends with the 'day students' and had the odd girlfriend, but nothing serious. There was lots of drinking, smoking and playing poker in the boarding house, and this was when I started smoking cigarettes, all in an effort to be one of the cool kids. The teasing stopped once I changed myself to fit in. I thought that being able to adapt to situations or adapt my personality to different people was a good thing, but I realise now that they didn't get to know the 'real me' and this began the toughest journey I've had of finding out who I really am. On a side note, I have since apologised to Dave for treating him the way I did at school, which he graciously accepted. I think noting that 'he knew', after all, he had been in the closet once too and knew how difficult accepting his own sexuality was.

At the beginning of my second year of boarding school, my parents split up. This was an interesting experience for me. I was happy for Mum and she seemed relieved. It was like a weight had been lifted off her shoulders. I remember her asking me, 'Do you think I made the right decision?' I didn't even need time to think before saying yes. I also felt a weird sense of relief within myself because I didn't enjoy being around Dad's depressed and angry moods and happy to now have the option to remove myself from that energy. However, I'll never forget the day Mum left Dad the letter to let him know the marriage was over. Talking about their marriage was not an option anymore for Mum as she had tried to get Dad to open up for years leading up to this, with no luck. I woke up one sunny Sunday morning after coming home from school for the weekend, I stumbled into the kitchen, Dad was sitting, moping as usual at the kitchen table. Mum must have been working, which she quite often did early on weekends to get out of the house and get on top of her busy workload. Dad sees me walk in and angrily mumbles, 'Your mother wants to break up.' Coincidentally, my seven-year-old sister arises from her bedroom and he tosses her the letter, then makes her read it out aloud. Quivering, she does her best to repeat the words written across the page. She was struggling, and the tears started to flow before reaching the end. I was shocked by Dad's actions. I watched him bounce between anger and sadness. He was in pain, and I have realised he wanted us to hurt as much as he was, to show us how much Mum had hurt him. That is a memory that will stay with me forever. I can't be angry at my dad for what he did on this day, all I can do is try to place myself in his shoes and understand why he made some poor choices that, perhaps, were part of the reason his relationship was ending that day.

The realisation

For as long as I can remember I have been attracted to boys. When I was about 12 years old, as the hormones began to rage, I realised that this attraction was only beginning to intensify. This is the age when boys begin fantasising about girls, yet whenever I masturbated as young boys do, I was always thinking of boys or searching on the internet for gay porn. I would go to a nearby town to buy gay magazines only to burn them all after looking at them as I felt so ashamed, and didn't want to get caught out by anyone. At boarding school, I began chatting to guys online – I'm unsure of how I managed to hide that in the dormitories. Somehow, I got a guy's number and we organised to meet up. I snuck out of the boarding house one night to meet him at the local lake where we hooked up in the back of the car, he was about 24 years old. I can still remember the intense smell of the leather seats in the back of his BMW. This was a nice experience; he was kind and not forceful, but I still felt sick afterwards. When I returned to the boarding house later that night, I cried in the shower, feeling so ill because of what I had done and so I deleted his number. Still feeling disgusted the next day, I continued to delete any matchmaking accounts that I had. I never saw him again, and don't even remember his name, as I felt so much shame. I repeated that pattern numerous times, this constant build-up of tension, a release and then the realisation of the shame surrounding my actions, until I came out. For so many years I was afraid of everything getting out of control and the truth exposing who I really was.

Coming out

Hiding my sexuality took a serious toll on me throughout high school. I so wanted to be able to be completely 'me', but instead I was a suppressed and tame version of myself. Somewhere along the line, I think one night when I was drunk, I told a friend that I was bisexual (which was a little closer to the truth). Kim was her name, and she was not my closest friend, but she had moved to Warracknabeal a couple years prior and because of this I felt safe enough to tell her. I think deep down I knew she would value our friendship more than outing me. After I left school, I attended a Rotary Youth Leadership Camp. The camp was for young people between the ages of 18 and 24 to learn how to be good leaders. Through lots of group activities over the week, we were forced to be vulnerable and ask ourselves tough questions to uncover the things that were holding us back. Basically, talking about stuff you don't normally talk about with people you hardly know. This experience definitely lit a fire in me to make some changes in my life. In order to find my truth, I felt I needed to move away from Warracknabeal and country Victoria – the big city was calling me. Melbourne was the place. I had dreamed about living in Melbourne ever since visiting for the first time as a kid. As a teenager, scouring the internet had made me realise that there were others like me in the big city, and I had dreamed of being in a bar with other gay men. Even though I was still (in my mind) a long way from coming out, I felt that by being around others like me was a start to understanding these feelings I had had since puberty. Once I had secured a basic barista job at Starbucks, I moved in with a family friend until I could find a proper place to live. I wasn't quite sure how that would happen. The family friend was a divorced, middle-aged ex-footballer who was quite macho. I didn't feel super comfortable with him, but it was just the situation I needed to motivate me to find another place. I was there for probably a month before I then moved in with someone I had met on the Rotary camp. One night I decided to go to a gay bar called The Exchange Hotel on Commercial Road in Prahran. Commercial Road used to be the place to go if you were a gay man in Melbourne, as there were gay bars, clubs and shops all along the strip and it was just around the corner from the infamous Chapel Street. This was big for me as I had only been to a gay bar once before, while underage, and it wasn't a very pleasurable experience. I was so drunk that I could barely remember the night (sorry, Mum). Not my finest moment, but I'm sure you can understand why. I started off with a few drinks at home then continued to drink by myself in a park behind the bar, just to get the courage to go in. Obviously, I was quite drunk by this stage, but I managed to pull it together enough to get in. In true gay bar style, there was a drag show on stage. As I was watching, feeling incredibly awkward and uncomfortable, I continued to drink at a faster-than-appropriate pace. With one arm on the bar pretending to look as cool as possible, this girl standing beside me started up a conversation. Her name was Lauren. She had just moved over from Tassie with her two best gay friends (Jarrod and Toni). She asked for my name and I responded with 'Jack'! I just blurted it out – Jack? Where had that come from? Will and Grace maybe? I was so nervous and still so unsure of whether I wanted to come out that I didn't want to be outed by a girl I barely knew. She ushered me to the smoking area so that we could hear each other better, and so I could meet the boys. The boys were super over the top, as camp as a row of tents, some may say, but what drew me to them was how absolutely comfortable they were with their sexuality. This meeting was a pivotal moment for me. We all exchanged numbers, and as our friendships blossomed over the coming weeks, so did my acceptance of my sexuality. I began to embrace my gayness and the gay community and felt so comfortable being around my new friends. I jumped in feet first and made the most of attending all the gay bars on offer – every weekend with my new friends was party weekend! It was absolutely liberating. At this stage, alcohol was the drug of choice, and my youthful age kept me bouncing back night after night. About a month into living my new double life, Mum came down to Melbourne for a work seminar and we planned dinner together. This was the night; I was going to come out. I wanted to tell her, and this was the opportunity to do so. She was alone and I knew this would be the last chance I would have for a while. I knew Mum wouldn't reject me, but there was still that little whisper in the back of my head, what if she did. I think all young gay kids will experience those thoughts. Now though, I had a group of friends to support me just in case. Sitting waiting for our entrée, my heart was pounding out of my chest, I could not keep calm, I was fidgety and restless. I looked at Mum and mumbled 'Mum, I think I have something to tell you.' She seemed concerned as she was not expecting this level of seriousness. Then I just burst out with, 'I'm gay.' As it turned out, Mum was amazing. We both cried as we held hands. I said to her, 'Surely you would have had some idea?' She said, 'No, I didn't.' I then went on to say, 'Even when I played with dolls with my female cousins and dressed up in girls' clothes and wigs with my sister?' to which she replied, 'I didn't think anything of it, you were just my son.' We continued to cry and laugh and drink our way through the meal. I had finally made the biggest decision of my life to this point – I had had my official 'coming out'. Not as dramatic as I had been so worried about, but the weight of the world had been lifted off my shoulders. I could finally begin to be the person I had been suppressing for all these years.

Mum decided she needed to tell the rest of my family back in the country, including Dad. Being a small town where the community thrives on gossip, she was worried that they would find out before I got a chance to tell them. I wish I had been strong enough to take that responsibility on myself, but I was still so vulnerable and agreed for her to do the deed. Fortunately, my family were very accepting which, again, was of great relief to me. My nan messaged me as soon as she had been told saying, 'Lindsay, we love you no matter what.'

Dad, on the other hand, was a different story. We weren't really that close at this point, so not hearing from him was not uncommon. He rang me at 3 am one Sunday morning when I had just finished working at this late-night pizza bar I had recently started at. Seeing his name pop up on my phone at 3 am induced immediate anxiety; I knew what he would be calling about. I was driving and so pulled over to answer the call. He was drunk. My memory is a little vague of the exact words he said, but I remember him asking me the question. 'So, Mum tells me you're gay?' My heart was pounding. 'Yes,' I responded. In his drunken state he proceeded to tell me that I shouldn't rush into these decisions and that it's probably just a phase. I said I'd been feeling this way for a while and that it was not a phase. I felt sick and very nervous having this conversation. I wanted to say so much more, but I was so scared. I wanted to tell him that I had been battling these feelings for years, and this decision to tell people about my sexuality was not a decision I had made lightly. Why would I put myself through this level of vulnerability, and open myself up to such rejection if it was not a serious thing? Being gay was still not such a socially accepted thing, so again, why would I openly allow for that rejection. My father had always intimidated me, and as he got older and his moodiness worsened, our connection fizzled. I had no more words, and to be honest having a serious conversation with him while he was so drunk was probably not the right time. This was the last time we spoke about my sexuality until I was 28.

13

Life after coming out

As I've expressed earlier, coming out lifted a huge weight off my shoulders. I remember describing it at the time as though the crushing weight of the world had been removed, and I could finally focus on something other than hiding a massive part of who I was. The reason this weight was so large was because while in hiding my sexuality, any type of effeminate tendency that would come through, I would suppress and force a level of masculinity that I knew was more accepted. Being so closeted and having so much resentment for the person that I had become, forced me to make calculating actions in all aspects of my life so as not to appear in any way gay. So, finally, I felt that I could be myself; I could embrace my femininity.

When I first came out, I certainly did embrace that suppressed femininity I had. It had been building up inside of me and came bursting out like a shaken-up bottle of soft drink. My new gay friends were owning it which gave me the courage to do the same. I was at every Kylie concert wearing glitter, I was experimenting with girls' clothes and wasn't afraid of a little bronzer and fake tan here and there. I succeeded in embracing gay culture by going to all the gay clubs, bars, dance parties and bookstores. I had finally accepted that I was gay, ready to open myself up to this new life. I was free to openly explore it without feeling that I could get caught out for doing something wrong. This was not possible for me in my hometown of Warracknabeal, and I was absolutely loving my new gay city life.

The first time I went home to Warracknabeal, about three months after coming out, was for Christmas, and I was petrified. My Christmas Eve tradition had always been about catching up with friends at the local pub and Christmas Day was about the family getting together. I had a couple of close friends that I went to the pub with that night, whom I had told prior that I was gay, but being a small town, I knew that everyone else at the pub would know, including some of my network of extended friends who I had not personally told. I was scared of how people would react; I had my guard well and truly up, ready to defend myself against any criticism or discrimination. I also knew that some of my high school bullies would be out and about, and who knows what they would have to say now that they were right about my sexuality. As it turned out, not one person said anything about me being gay at all! I think between not having the confidence to bring it up and probably having some inclination anyway, everyone just avoided the topic, but at the same time treated me as if nothing had happened. It was the best outcome that I would never have even imagined. The walls I had barricaded myself with were not needed. I actually ended up in tears at one point, overjoyed with the acceptance I had felt from my home community. It was an amazing feeling!

Ultimately, hiding for so long and internalising the homophobia I had experienced left me struggling to find who I really was. Coming out was just the first step of a long and tumultuous journey to self-acceptance and love.

Influences in search of happiness

Throughout my life I have struggled to find a male role model who embraced his masculinity with empathy and compassion. I did not find this in my father nor in the other older males around me. I was different to other boys, and in my search for the perfect male role model I came to realise there is no such thing. I've consequently been influenced by many people in my life, some of whom have only been around for a short time, and others for a long time. The culmination of these influences has helped me to heal over the years, taking bits and pieces from every person that I meet.

A few that come to mind have shown me what is achievable when you work hard and focus your attention inward to discover what's personally holding you back. For example, one of my friends, who has been around the party scene with me, has shown me what it takes to crawl out of the self-suffocating space of substance misuse. I witnessed his journey of sobriety. He always had a natural ability to be the centre of attention; his charisma is palpable and he spent most of his early twenties couch surfing and partying. Watching him, I realised what he was doing to himself and just how much more amazing he is sober, was awe inspiring to me. He is one of those people who actually doesn't need to use a drug for confidence or courage – he is bloody brilliant without it. He is talented and brings an amazing energy to every person he comes into contact with. Watching this friend battle his demons and consciously change his path, was the first time I had seen someone turn their life around and it gave me the courage to do the same.

There is another person in my network who has shown me that changing your trajectory in life at any age is possible. He used to be a hospitality worker like me and around the age of 30 he started studying. As each year passed, I felt like my opportunity to study and change my career path was slipping away. Watching someone else tread the road similar to mine, helped me see a path I didn't know existed later in life, and I thank him for that.

Each person in my life challenges me, this is something I have only recently realised. I think that getting older has been a blessing in understanding my place in the world, and the types of people and influences I need around me. Not everyone possesses the most positive characteristics but that is something that I have learnt to live with. Some friends and family teach me how I don't want to be; a valuable insight that takes maturity to understand. Others influence me to be the best version of myself through their actions, as I see them challenging themselves, constantly learning, growing and displaying those authentic characteristics I'm so drawn to. Overall, I think my biggest influence has been my higher self. Through self-reflection, self-gratification and some honest truths, I have been able to overcome many obstacles and I am super proud of myself for that.

Biggest challenges in life

I think every gay man has some tough challenges to overcome throughout his life. Just the simple fact of feeling the need to 'come out' is challenge enough that nearly all gay men will face. My first biggest challenge has been managing my relationship with my dad. I would love to have a more wholesome and honest relationship with him, but that just doesn't seem to be possible. I wish I was strong enough within myself to be able deflect his negativity, but I am too sensitive and can't help but internalise those feelings. I struggle with the way he reacts to me as I can see now that he doesn't have the emotional intelligence to deal with life. I don't think he's capable of conversing with me on any level other than everyday surface stuff. He rarely asks me anything about my life. I hear him use self-sabotaging language, and he doesn't have enough self-worth to be able to pull down his own walls and be a father for me. When I reflect on his behaviour, I'm not sure if he will ever be able to build on our relationship, or want to, and this may be something that I am going to have to continue to work on myself. His personal history growing up has led him to be the person he is today, and I can't change that. I am entering a place where I'm gaining the courage and conviction to move on with my own life knowing that until he chooses to work on himself, we may never have the father/son relationship that I have desperately craved. I bounce between that thought and the thought that if I continue to work on myself, I may have the strength to be able to deflect his negativity and be content with what relationship we have. I am definitely in a place where I don't judge him for his incapacity to connect with me, I accept that he is who he is, but I am still struggling to understand how I feel about the relationship that we have. Unfortunately for my dad, his disconnection from his mental health has cost him a relationship with his family and his homophobia has led to a fractured and disjointed relationship with his son. The cost to me has been (the lack of) a positive male role model. I hope that this isn't always the case, and that one day I can be proud of the relationship my dad and I have.

The second major challenge for me has been suffering from confusing and restricting mental health issues which led to a very unhealthy relationship with drugs. My mental health began to decline around the age of 13 as I started to realise that I wasn't like the other boys. As I've mentioned, I displayed more feminine tendencies or was not as 'masculine' as the other boys, and as I lived in a country town, these tendencies were viewed as abnormal, or more frankly, in their words, gay. I started getting teased about being gay which was extremely hurtful. Being gay was seen as bad or wrong – definitely not acceptable. This was evident through language, such as, 'That's gay', relating to something being negative or when someone would say, 'That's a bit gay, isn't it?', inferring that it was wrong to be gay. As I battled with the realisation that I was gay, so did

I have to grapple with my internal struggle and the teasing I faced. I didn't want to be gay, I wanted to be like everyone else. My understanding of 'gay', was instilled in me by society and my peers that it was a bad thing, and why would I choose to be bad. This led me to throw all my energy into other areas of my life, studying, working (I used to run a little pamphlet delivery business around town), then into unhealthy habits like binge eating. The binge eating stayed with me for years and has been something I have only been able to work on properly over the past 12 months. Consequently, I have struggled with my weight and being overweight for most of my life has added to my ill mental health.

As I reached a less frowned-upon drinking age, 15, I turned my bingeing nature towards alcohol. As I mentioned before, I started drinking and smoking while I was at boarding school to fit in with the heterosexual boys. As my reliance on vices increased, my grades dropped. I went from an A-grade student to somewhere in the middle. Drinking numbed the pain of hiding my true identity, and smoking made me feel as though I was part of a community. Being a teenager and a smoker, you are part of a small underground network of people who you become close with for the mere fact you all share the same secret. These coping strategies only intensified as I got older.

Once I moved to Melbourne and had officially come out, I found some sort of happiness. I think being openly gay was the release I needed, as I felt free to be me. I started making friends as the new me and they were exciting times. But not dealing with some of the trauma of being closeted would come back to haunt me. At the age of 21, I was introduced to methamphetamine (ice) and although I don't blame the drug for the next few rollercoaster years, an emotionally numbing drug like ice has the power to attach itself to a vulnerable and unstable young adult like myself. Within six months of my first exposure to ice, I was using every day. I went from being a valuable employee to one that struggled to find clarity and meaning, with my mental health spiralling out of control. I was so scared of what was happening to me. I couldn't understand why I needed to use all the time, so I made the decision to move back home to Warracknabeal with my mum to get clean. At the time, I thought I just had a drug issue, not realising it was actually a psychological problem. By moving home, I was really just running away from the problems in my mind. My poor mum didn't know what to do and tried so hard to understand and help me heal, but the next three years turned out to be the toughest on my mental and physical health. In this three-year period, I felt extremely claustrophobic in Warracknabeal as I had no friends with common interests, and less freedom than I did in Melbourne. I really missed being able to dance at a club, catch up with my friends and by this point I had been dabbling in the art of DJing, but this was not a culturally popular artform in a country town. At 21, the small-town mentality was not for me. I felt extremely vulnerable because of my drug use, underlying mental health and being back in the country made me feel very exposed to the judgement from others. The only difference in my drug habit once moving home was that I used at every opportunity rather than every day. So, I never achieved the intended goal of getting clean, which was a lesson I had to learn in order to dig beneath the surface of the addiction.

Three years in the country and I had had enough. What prompted me to move back to Melbourne was the realisation that I wasn't going to find happiness in Warracknabeal at that time, and the opportunity to meet any fellow gay counterparts or future lovers in the country was slim. I was 24 when I returned to Melbourne. I was in quite a good headspace as I was excited about moving back and connecting with new friends I'd been building from a distance. I was exercising and eating well, healthy habits that I had tended to neglect in the past. This only lasted for a few months before the substance use crept back into my life. I was managing a late-night venue, and this time, the use was gradual and over the course of three years it snuck back into every element of my life. It was my secret. Most people around me didn't know the extent that I was abusing my body with narcotics. By the age of 25, I was back using ice every day, and this continued for quite some time. The difference this time was that I was older, and I'd been down this path before, so it wasn't as scary for me. I kept trying to convince myself that while I still had a job and somewhat in control, I could continue using. Over time, this became increasingly more difficult. For starters, it was becoming harder to fund my growing habit. I was convinced that I was functioning at 100 per cent, yet looking back my behaviour was so erratic.

When I was 27, with a daily ice habit, my world was turned upside down. One day I was driving home from work, having lost my licence the week before for losing 12 demerit points, when I was pulled over by the Police. I was shitting bricks! I had a whole chemist of drugs in my car as I'd been dealing to fund my growing addiction. The cops, after realising I had no licence, decided to search my car, where they found my stash of drugs that I wasn't very clever at concealing. At this point they handcuffed me, threw me to the ground and their whole attitude towards me changed. They pushed me into the back of the divvy van, and off we went to the police station where they proceeded to search me for further drugs. They led me to a tiny windowless room where one officer forced me to take every piece of clothing off my body, I was then told to squat and cough to check whether I had any drugs in my anal cavity. This was one of the most humiliating experiences of my life. I felt like my world was crashing down before my eyes, as each minute passed the realisation that I'd let down my family and myself was becoming evident. As I stood there shivering in my birthday suit, any thought of a positive life was slipping away. I was questioned for hours, and my phone was confiscated along with any money and drugs that they had found. By 5 am the next morning, I left the police station, charged with possession of multiple drugs and some in a trafficable quantity.

For a few weeks after that I tried to get clean, but to no avail. I was in too deep, and the pending court case was only adding to my heightened levels of depression and anxiety that I just couldn't face. Until one day when I bumped into friend who was a lawyer, and she gave me the best basic advice on what to do to help my cause. She said, 'It's time to work out your shit!', and gave me some suggestions on how to do that but could not tell me from experience what exactly was going to work. However, having someone believe in me was enough to take some affirmative action. Firstly, I researched free drug addiction facilities as I didn't have money to pay for rehabilitation. I was not ready to tell my family what had happened, as I was so ashamed that I was back in an even worse position than I was when I had moved back home with Mum to Warracknabeal.

I ended up attending a free detox program at a public health unit called, Wellington House. My research also led me to find a six-week group therapy for gay men who use ice called Re-Wired at Thorne Harbour Health. I started seeing a psychologist-in-training which was covered under Medicare, as well as attending many Narcotics Anonymous meetings. This immersion in multiple forms of therapy was critical to my recovery. It was a process that required me to be surrounded by positive influences, that forced me to turn inward and understand the reasons I was self-medicating with ice. This was only the beginning of my recovery though, and I continued to support my wellness journey by seeing a clinical psychologist who specialises in drug and alcohol and LGBTIQ issues. As I now know, it was battling with my identity and the heteronormative experiences of growing up that were behind some of my drug use, masking my feelings of not being accepted by others and myself.

I'm pleased to say that my day in court eight months later turned out much better than I imagined. The result was a Community Correction Order which meant that if I committed another offense within the following 18 months, I may very well have ended up in jail. I also had to perform 100 hours of community work within the next 12 months with regular drug testing being part of the conditions. I finished my 100 hours community work in seven months and returned to Court to request the Community Correction Order be revoked, and to my delight it was. That was the last shedding of my rocky past. I do believe that the hard work I put in to rehabilitate myself created the more lenient outcome. As I was talking to Anne about my story, I realised I passed a milestone of 900 days clean, and I couldn't be prouder of myself for this achievement.

I am now 31, and the past four years since that sliding doors moment of sitting naked in a police station have been anything but easy. My recovery journey has not just been about stopping my ice use, it has been about understanding why I was self-medicating with a powerful stimulant to numb me from the pain of depression. My journey has taught me that I will always have to be aware of what choices I make in life, that will have positive and negative effects on my mental health. I am not cured and may never be, but I am okay with that. I am now the happiest and most authentic version of myself. I have explored, through therapy and lots of self-reflection that I could never meet up to the mountainous standards I had set for myself to feel worthy enough of acceptance. I am who I am, I am worthy of love and I am accepted. A by-product has also been delving into the unhealthy relationship I had with food, and since this realisation, I have become fit, healthy and I enjoy putting my mind and body first. Finding my authentic self is a journey and one on which I now embrace the ups and downs. There's no end goal, it is simply about enjoying the process and being grateful for every day I have on this planet.

What would you tell your younger self?

What I realised through my challenging experiences is that to be my authentic self, I had to wade through the quagmire of crappy emotions to find the real me and this takes time, effort and courage. I think even more so for gay men than our heterosexual peers. I needed a clear mind before I could really work out who I am and what I stand for. Reflecting on my past mistakes has enabled me to search for authenticity and accept those flaws that have actually helped me to be more grounded, happier and educated. I am grateful for my experiences. I am now studying social work to enhance my understandings of the world and my place in it, and without these past experiences, I would perhaps never have realised that this is the path I'm meant to be on.

Therefore, I would tell my younger self to celebrate the person you are right now including all your flaws and accept them as making up the unique person you are. People love you for who you are, so don't be afraid to be yourself. I can't say don't do this or don't do that because that never stopped me from making plenty of, ultimately rewarding, mistakes to learn from. You will experience much adversity in your life, and that will shape the beautiful man you will become. For me, my past addiction does not define me; it is proof that I am strong and resilient enough to overcome a massive challenge and am capable of achieving all the things I want to. I truly am worthy of love and so are you.

Kevin

The younger years

King Island is a beautiful island off the south coast of Adelaide that is well known for its high-quality beef and dairy products. I was born into a farming family that ran a dairy farm on King Island providing milk for the King Island Butter company. I have three brothers and three sisters and, as you can imagine, living on a remote island has its challenges as everyone knows your business and life was quite sheltered. Myself and my siblings attended King Island High School while Dad ran the dairy farm and Mum tended to the family, Dad enjoyed a drink with his mates (at times too much), and on occasion the responsibility of looking after the dairy fell on to the children. It was a tough life.

Football was one of the few sports played on the island and my brothers and father loved the game, both playing and watching. However, my favourite game was not football, it was one that I played with my sister, Bernadette. We had a lovely long porch on either side of the house, that we would line up with lots of dolls and teddy bears. I would take great delight in dressing up in my mother's high heel shoes, a petticoat for a dress and pretend to serve the dolls and bears their inflight meals and drinks. We could play that for hours, then my mother would come out and say, 'Kev, your dad's about to come in through the front gate, get out of those clothes and pack up!' I played this delightful game up to the age of 12 years old. Another fond memory I have is with my mum. There were times when I would arrive home from school, and Mum would insist that I dance with her around the lounge room as she jitterbugged to In the Mood by Glen Miller. This opened my eyes to the love of dancing and how free it made me feel. Then as I got older, I loved go-go dancing to music at home, much to my father's frustration and eye rolling. I'm sure he wondered at times if I was really his son.

My dad came home one day when I was 16 years old and said, 'I've got a job for you! You can board in Melbourne with your sister and brother-in-law, as they've got a job for you at Simmons Bedding Co.' There was no discussion about this massive change to my life, as it was an order, but to be honest, I was just happy to get off the island, especially to Melbourne. So, a couple of weeks later I was at the airport with my mum and dad, with case in hand. My dad declared to me as I was about to board the plane, 'Alright son, all the best, look after yourself and don't write home for money because you won't get it!' Then he shook my hand as a goodbye. That was the best he had to offer! From that day, I made a pact with myself, at the tender age of 16, to never ask for money. I moved in with my sister and brother-in-law where I paid $13 board per week that came out of my wage of $46 per week.

And so, the fun began! By now it was the early seventies, and lifestyles in Melbourne compared to King Island were worlds apart as I felt so free in Melbourne away from prying eyes. One of my favourite clubs to visit was called Sweethearts in St Kilda. Here I would go-go dance for free drinks. It was like a dream come true to get free drinks for something that I loved to do.

At this stage, I still hadn't officially come out as it was not widely accepted. There was also a bit of denial going on. So much so, that when I was 20 years old, I started dating a girl called Josephine. We were together for two years with talk of getting engaged, when I realised I couldn't deny any longer that I was definitely gay. I had finally accepted that it was men that I loved, not women. Even through that two-year period, I continued to have flings with other men, so it was the right thing to do for both our sakes. I tried to let Josephine down as gently as possible. I was really trying to do the right thing in straight society, but I couldn't lie to myself anymore.

The realisation

I think the first inkling that I was gay was at the age of 11 or 12 years old. When watching television in the early seventies, there was a show called Magnum PI with Tom Selleck as the main character. I thought he was the most gorgeous man I had ever seen, and even then, I fantasised about being his boyfriend. I always enjoyed playing female roles which led to me being the more feminine person in my relationships.

At the age of 15, I fancied a boy at school who was a year above me. This is when I first acted on the feelings of being gay, as I went on to have an affair with him. Our first fling happened in the locker room at school – I know, not so romantic. However, this experience did not cement for me the fact that I was gay, and I continued to stay in the closet as I was more worried about my father finding out, especially if he was on a drinking binge with his mates.

Coming out

I was officially outed to my parents by one of my sisters when I was 24 years old. She rang me one day and said, 'I've told Mum and Dad that you're gay. Dad said he's fine with it and Mum said there are doctors that can help him with that!' This was Mum's strict Catholic upbringing kicking in, but to her credit, she didn't really harp on it and accepted me for who I am. So, as it turned out, there wasn't as big a 'hoo-hah' as I thought there would be. Having said that, I was really more annoyed with my sister for exposing me like that, as she had no right! Even after officially coming out though, I still was having trouble accepting the fact that I was gay. A friend referred me to a wonderful doctor who set me straight (pardon the pun). This doctor sat me down and basically said, 'What are you worried about the most?' I replied, 'I'm still worried about what my father would think as he is a tough man with old fashioned views.' The doctor replied with, 'It's your life and you live it the way you want to live it, it has nothing to do with anyone else!' Just hearing those words helped to open my eyes to a better life, and I floated out the doctor's office and continued to live my life on my terms.

Life after coming out

I felt more positive about myself and as though a burden had been lifted as I didn't have to live a lie anymore. I could be who I wanted to be, and felt more content knowing who I am and happier within myself. I firstly had to accept the fact that I was gay before I could feel comfortable about it. Generally, my family accepted the news. They never brought it up and life went on as normal. I was one of the lucky ones in that my family did not reject me, seeing that it was in the seventies when I came out. I do feel that the belief I have in myself as a person is why I have never felt ashamed of who I am.

I have a drink coaster with a saying on it that relates to my name and I think it sums me up:

Kevin

From the Gaelic meaning 'gentle'.

He is youthful and fun, friendly and kind, but has a stubborn streak.

He sticks to his principles.

I believe these principles, and possibly my stubborn streak, have kept me sane and able to face the challenges that have come my way.

Influences in search of happiness

As the years rolled on, so did my weight. I was in a relationship with my partner, Andrew, for 37 years and fell into the role of the wife. Very clichéd, I know. I looked after the running of the house and our lives while Andrew went to work, making it a very traditional household like my parents. I became content and complacent in this relationship. I stopped looking after myself, resulting in me leading an incredibly unhealthy lifestyle of no exercise and plenty of junk food.

One day, Andrew announced (quite offhandedly) that he was having an affair with a boy that was 35 years younger. I was in shock and felt like I'd been slapped in the face. This was a huge wake up call for me. After the breakup, I realised how much I had let myself go. I had an appointment at my doctors where I was promptly told that I needed to lose weight as I had type 2 diabetes and was on the verge of being dependent on insulin. Later that day, I was sitting in a café sipping on a cappuccino and eating banana bread, feeling very sorry for myself. I looked up and saw a sign for a local personal training studio called Vision and the owner, David, was sitting there speaking to potential clients. I made a decision to check it out, and turned my life around! That was four years ago. I'm now 40 kg lighter, stronger and healthier than I've ever been in my life. Banana bread no longer passes these lips, and my emotional health is much improved since deciding to put myself first, and appreciate the body I've been given. I now stand up for myself and value who I am. It's only taken 65 years, but better late than never.

Biggest challenges in life

I had a few blokes at my workplace over the years ask me if I was gay, to which I replied 'Yes.' There would be some sniggering and sometimes they even backed away from me as if I was a threat. I would say to them, 'I wouldn't want you, I prefer real men!' Their reactions always amazed me, as they were incensed as though it were a dent to their ego even though they were straight. However, as time went on, some actually became my protectors. If anyone targeted me about being gay when at the pub after work having drinks with the boys, they were very quick to defend me. I think because I didn't hide the fact, there was no ammunition to throw back at me. Looking back at that time, I realise now that by standing up for myself and not hiding that I was gay, took the sting out of their prejudices.

One of my biggest challenges in life has been supporting my ex-partner, Andrew, who is now an alcoholic. I love him dearly as a friend and to watch him battle his demons is extremely hard. He's never told me what's behind his personal struggles and he doesn't want to talk about it, which at times is very frustrating. I've had to learn to live my own life and support him the best way I can without compromising who I am. I can't help but think, that his alcoholism is due to him not coming out until he was 30 years old. Even when he did finally come out to his parents they were in total denial, to the point where his mother would continue to suggest suitable girlfriends. I imagine this would have had a profound impact on him in relation to accepting himself and being good enough in his Parents' eyes.

What would you tell your younger self?

When opportunity knocks, answer the door! This will allow you to follow your dreams and ambitions. I regret not finding the courage to become a drag queen. I always loved to dress up and dance, especially in high shoes or boots, miniskirts, tight tops and wigs. When I was in my mid-twenties I would go to gay clubs dressed up in drag for a bit of fun. One night, a girlfriend asked if I and my friends would dress up in drag as entertainment at her 21st birthday party. This inspired me to audition as a drag queen at the George Hotel on Fitzroy Street, St Kilda. I was so nervous when I arrived. After being introduced to the producer of the shows, Art Luden, I was taken out the back where I was provided with a costume and had my makeup done. I was dressed in a tight pink dress with spaghetti straps, pink stilettos, sixties black wig and stunning makeup. I felt fabulous and was in my element – I loved it! I lip-synced to You Only Live Twice by Nancy Sinatra. I knew my audition was successful as I could hear Art clapping when I finished, and then he said, 'Kevin, I want you to think hard on this, because I think you've got potential and we can use you in the show.' I was so happy until I could hear my father's words of disapproval in my head. I felt it would be difficult to go back home to King Island feeling ashamed of being a drag queen. In hindsight, he would have coped with me being a drag queen, but I didn't want to embarrass him. So, to this day, I regret that I never gave it a chance.

Another regret I have is not pursuing a career as an interior designer. I have been told over the years that I have an eye for styling houses. When I was in my late thirties, I had already decorated four properties that I lived in, and a friend of mine suggested that I have a flare for decorating, and that I should get a qualification to take it up as a career. At that time, I didn't have a driver's licence and it would have taken me at least three hours each day to travel to and from school. I wish I had not let that inconvenience put me off my passion. Having said that, now at the age of 65 and more time on my hands, there's nothing to stop me from becoming an interior stylist so all is not lost.

My motto is the Nike slogan – Just Do It!

Nathan

The younger years

I grew up as an only child in the beautiful seaside town of Terrigal in New South Wales where I attended Central Coast Grammar School. My parents had both been married before they met and were flight attendants with the same airline. As a child, I loved to perform for family and friends and would often be dressed up in my mum's clothes to entertain the visitors through various artforms. This came naturally to me, enabling me to express myself as an entertainer and tap into my flamboyant side. This behaviour was not considered unusual in my household, as my parents had many gay friends through their work who frequently visited our home, so I knew they were very open-minded.

The realisation

I remember quite vividly when I was seven years old, the film Titanic was the latest blockbuster. After watching this movie, I woke up in the middle of the night to then go and wake my mum up to speak with her. I went on to tell her that I thought I was gay because I was attracted to Leonardo DiCaprio, rather than Kate Winslet. Mum listened to me intently, then we went on to have a discussion about how it's okay to like who you like. The way she said it, in her caring manner, reassured me that no matter the outcome, I was loved. So, off I wandered not really thinking too much more about it. It was in Year 6 that I realised I was definitely more attracted to men but continued to suppress those feelings. I'd had the odd crush on girls in primary school, but they never eventuated to a romance which meant that I never really explored that aspect of my sexuality. The internal battle over my sexuality continued until Year 11. By that point, I couldn't ignore who I was any longer, and this outweighed my fear of coming out, and possibly of being rejected for being different from everyone else.

Coming out

Whilst I had been experimenting discussing my sexuality with people online throughout Year 11, it wasn't until Year 12 that I felt comfortable enough to come out to one of my best friends. This eventuated after a night of drinking and dancing at a friend's 18th birthday, as she casually slipped into our conversation, asking me if I was gay. My intoxication gave me a little bit of extra courage which, mixed with the casualness of her question, helped me get over the line and admit to her that I thought I was bisexual. We chatted a bit, and I felt relief that I had finally told someone who was close to me that was extremely supportive. Over the next six-month period, I began to tell my closest friends. At the same time, there was plenty going on at home as my grandmother, who lived with us, was very ill, and I felt it wasn't the right time to drop that bombshell on my parents.

Once my grandmother had passed, I decided it was time to tell them the news. The night in question was not planned at all; it was a last-minute decision. I marched up the stairs to where my parents were watching television and announced that I had something to tell them. Consequently, the television was put on mute and there was no turning back. I then proceeded to proclaim that I was gay. My dad laughed and said, 'Tell us something we don't know!', and Mum said, 'I've been trying to coax it out of you over the past few weeks, especially with the friends you've been bringing home.' Who would have thought all that worry was for nothing? I sat down and we chatted some more. They told me how much they loved me and being gay did not change how they felt about me. I felt a huge sense of relief once my parents knew.

I believe the saying 'the truth will set you free', and that's exactly how it felt after coming out. Accepting myself for being gay was the hardest part, and then having to tell my parents, but thankfully taking those brave steps was worth it.

None of my close friends and family had any issue with me being gay, so I was fortunate that I didn't directly experience homophobia. However, the first time I had to deal with homophobia was through my first boyfriend whose family did not accept their son as gay. Consequently, we had to sneak around to see each other, and I wasn't used to that, making me feel like I was back in the closet. I wouldn't recommend sneaking around as it's not a healthy way to live, in fact, it's tiring as you're always looking over your shoulder trying to not get caught.

Life after coming out

When I was 19, I moved to Melbourne and met a group of people who took me under their wing and introduced me to the gay lifestyle. They were people of all ages, which is quite common in the gay community. I had finally found my tribe that I could relate to and didn't have to explain myself. They just got me! They showed me a world of beauty and fun, including taking party drugs every weekend which heightened my sense of freedom. They were successful, intelligent people, and there were no explanations needed as we were all the same. I was able to embrace the gay lifestyle and be part of a community, rather than feeling like someone on the outer, like I did growing up.

After a couple of years in Melbourne I moved back home to Terrigal for about six months to have a little break from my hectic life, after which I then moved to Sydney when I was 21. I began a relationship with a boyfriend who was 11 years my senior. I was a bit lost at that stage and this boyfriend helped to give me some stability after my partying ways in Melbourne. I decided to become a flight attendant and while training, broke up with my boyfriend. The lifestyle of a flight attendant for me, was like living a champagne life on a beer budget, as I partied my way around the world while working – at that stage, life was all about having fun!

Influences in search of happiness

My parents have been a huge influence in my life. At the age of 27, Mum found out she couldn't get pregnant due to endometriosis. She met my dad at 33 and fell pregnant with me at the age of 35, which was a miracle. While pregnant she had a car accident and fell down a set of stairs, yet I still survived. At 37 years old, Mum had lots of health issues and required a hysterectomy, but her specialist at the time strongly advised her that it wasn't necessary. Mum had to insist that she wanted to have it done and he finally gave in. After the operation, the specialist came into the ward with an ashen face and told her that if she hadn't had the operation, she would have died within the next two months due to cancer. With everything that Mum and Dad had gone through, they really have lived life to the fullest and are in love with each other to this day. Their love for each other and outlook on life has inspired me to have a relationship with a partner that emulates my parents.

When I was 22, I had an on/off relationship over a three-and-a-half-year period with a guy named Ryan who was 11 years my senior. As he was older than me, I was constantly surrounded by older people who definitely had a positive influence on me due to their various life experiences. The first time Ryan and I broke up it was like the end of the world for me; I was so dramatic and immature about it. As time went on with a few more bumps in the road of our relationship, we finally agreed it wasn't working. Instead of all the dramatics as in the past, I accepted the decision and was able to move on with the next chapter of my life. This relationship I would credit as helping me to mature and realise my self-worth, and I am forever grateful to Ryan.

My current relationship is with Wade, who I've been with for five years. I'm pleased to say that our relationship is as strong as my parents', and I consider myself very fortunate to have met him. He's taught me to be calmer and more grounded by not stressing as much. He's a great listener, makes me feel loved and supported and keeps me challenged by holding me accountable to my goals. This has allowed me to continue to grow within our relationship, so I don't feel I'm lost with who I am. I do believe that my previous relationships have all taught me something about myself, so when Wade appeared in my life, I was ready to settle down.

Biggest challenges in life

The hardest period in my life is the year I came out, as I lost not only my grandmother who lived with us, but also two grandfathers and my father's best friend who was like an uncle to me. While coming to terms with coming out that year, I coped by suppressing my grief over the loss of my loved ones which lead to a depressive couple of years. I was a bit lost and didn't know what to do with my life, so I filled it in with partying, drugs and hedonistic lifestyle. I was never fully addicted, but really loved the fun I had whilst taking drugs. Once I met Wade, I realised he was that 'special someone' I wanted in my life. He said that he wasn't really happy about my partying ways, particularly in relation to drugs. Even though, at the time, I couldn't really see the problem or where it could lead, I agreed to stop using them. It was around this time I started on the path of spirituality that has now influenced my whole life, and has strongly influenced my career, as I'm now a kinesiologist.

My other challenge, which I am still working on, is what goes on in my own head as I'm my own worst enemy. I've had very little external resistance in my life. However, my biggest struggles are all self-inflicted about how I think I should be, not who I am. Even with all the knowledge and tools I use as a kinesiologist, I still manage to get caught up in my own negative thoughts about myself. As the saying goes, 'Life is a journey and there's no real end goal.'

What would you tell your younger self?

I have an analogy that I'd like to give. Society sets certain expectations for us to fulfil in order to be happy. It's like being on a racetrack where everyone is racing around the same traditional track – it's paved, neat and tidy and everyone knows their place. But when you come out, you're not on the same track anymore. You've come off the traditional track and now find yourself racing through the bushes and onto the grass where it's much harder to navigate. The rules are different now, but if you can accept the change, it can be quite liberating. You can now run your own race without having to follow society's rules, and you can exist outside those traditional expectations. You can just be you. There would be no more questions about when you are going to meet a nice girl and settle down; it's more acceptable to be a little quirky or different. You've given up your right to run around the traditional racetrack, but you can have adventures without the weight of traditional society on your shoulders.

I would like to tell my younger self to worry less and stress less, however I don't think my younger self would hear that. You have to go through your trials and tribulations to heal, grow and develop as a person, so that you can accept the over thinking and challenging times knowing that you'll get through them. Take note of the people that surround you and see yourself though your family and friends' eyes, as that is who you really are. Don't let the misconceptions you have about yourself get in the way of your own happiness.

Peter

The younger years

I grew up during the 1960s and 1970s in a busy household with my mum, dad, three brothers and three sisters. We lived in a small, three-bedroom home in a south-east suburb of Melbourne, Victoria. I was the youngest in the family, and until I was seven years old, slept in my parents' room as there was no space left in the other two bedrooms until my eldest brother moved out. Life was great growing up with so many siblings because I had built-in playmates! I also had all the kids in the street to play with so there was plenty of fun to be had. Family life was everything to me.

We were a good, practising Catholic family, attending Catholic schools, and participating in many of the Parish events, actively playing sport for the school teams and participating in youth group activities. My parents went to church every week and even though they were religious, it was the social aspect that appealed to them the most. Mum and Dad often entertained the nuns and priests with a meal and drinks together on Sunday nights, making it normal for us to be surrounded by religious people.

Once I left school, I decided to become a primary school teacher, where I trained at a campus of the Catholic University of Melbourne. I had a good career with plenty of opportunities for leadership positions, eventually reaching high level positions in the Catholic education system as Principal and Team Leader in various system offices around Australia. There is no doubt that this work shaped my personal and professional decisions along the way, because when I reflect on it now, I was involved in the Catholic schooling system, as a student, or educator from 1970 to 2014. It is fairly obvious that the 44 years of living within that culture would influence my thoughts and ideas about myself and the world.

My personal goals revolved, almost solely, around having my own family. My memories of my own family growing up, were so positive that I wanted to recreate them in my own. I actually met my 'future wife' at university, although we were only friends at first. It wasn't an instant love affair, more a mutual respect and enjoyment of each other's company that would lead us to get married. I remember sitting in the car one night after we had been out with a group of friends, no doubt we were laughing over something funny, but we ended up looking at each other and agreeing that because we were such good friends, we should get married. The idea of marrying my best friend seemed a wonderful idea. So, we did. In the coming years, that friendship was to be greatly tested, and unfortunately wouldn't withstand the strain of later events that would challenge and change us forever.

Only in retrospect, from where I am now, can I see that I censored myself for many years before I came out. Some of you may smirk, or even laugh, at that idea, but I truly didn't think I was gay at the time. It is true that I avoided friends who might think I was gay and conversations about being gay, but that was more out of not wanting to appear gay rather than being found out. I grew up in a homophobic culture, reinforced by the people around me often making disparaging comments about gay people and their community. Often when I reflect on my growing up years, I cannot honestly remember meeting anyone that was openly gay. The people in my suburb, who were labelled gay, were often effeminate and because of that, were teased and harassed with incredible viciousness. For me, I wasn't effeminate, (although when I revisit some photos of me as a kid, I laugh about the fact that it was debatable!) and I wasn't going to put myself in a position that attracted such appalling behaviour from friends and family. I just didn't want to be gay.

I do remember constantly watching how I spoke, how I laughed and what I said, in case someone called me out for being gay. I would always have two conversations going on in my head at the same time to make sure I didn't say anything that would give me away. Perhaps no one would have guessed, or if they did, they wouldn't have cared, but I was hypersensitive to my behaviour because I did not want to be gay! Pure and simple, but at the same time, difficult and complex!

Having two conversations going on in my head at all times was exhausting, but that was not the only thing going on. I remember how, for many years, I also had this 'white noise' in my head, like the old sound televisions or radios made when they are not tuned into a proper channel. I lived with this noise for many, many years, not realising that it was perhaps caused by the confusion in my head that I would not admit to. Interestingly, on the day I came out, the 'white noise' ceased.

I had a similar experience with shoulder pain. About 12 months before I came out, my shoulder started aching to the point where I sought medical assistance. Often, I would sit at tables and hold my arm up so that I would not put weight on my shoulder. My shoulder would feel as if it was pulling out if its socket with excruciating pain. The physiotherapist that I visited, was booking me in twice a week and attempted everything to ease the pain. She became as frustrated as I was when the pain continued over the year. Surprisingly, or in hindsight, the pain ceased the day I admitted to myself that I was gay. I have not experienced that pain again! It's amazing how the body reacts to stress and then changes as the source of the stress is reduced or eliminated.

The realisation

With hindsight, I could go back to the age of around 12 years old and see the signs that I was gay. I do remember having pictures of half-naked men in my desk drawer, hidden from view, that would only come out when no one was home. I often fantasised about guys and bought magazines that had a male centrefold. I am not sure of how I explained these types of activities to myself as I was growing up, but remember justifying to myself that it was okay. Once I closed the drawer, or put the magazine away, those feelings were also packed away. I went back to being Peter and no one knew that I had those thoughts because they too were packed away. This ability to open part of my life, then close it and move on, was to become my way of dealing with the growing realisation that I was gay.

I would often put myself in situations where I could potentially meet men. I ran to keep fit. When running I would run to a beach that was a well-known meeting place for gay men. At first, I didn't know this, but when I found out I kept returning. I started using my second name as an alter ego if I met anyone at the beach. When the time was up, and I needed to go home, I turned my back on the beach and the guys I had met, much like closing the drawer or putting the magazine away. Always there came a time that I went back to being Peter and rejoined my family.

My family life was wonderful. My kids were then, and still are, the most important thing in my life. I have two handsome sons and a gorgeous daughter whom I adore. They made being Peter more important than being James – the alter ego I adopted. It was my middle name and I would use it when I needed to take time out from my so-called 'straight life'. It was easy to put James back in the drawer and return to my family, as they made my life wonderful.

In my late thirties, I struck up a friendship with a guy I had met at the beach. He became a very good friend and we regularly went for coffees or beers. Over time, I began to be introduced to his friends and we started to become very close. After a while, this friend, knowing that I was married and had children said, 'I can't do this anymore.' The friendship we had was platonic, but it hurt when this friendship was taken away from me. I couldn't or didn't want to see it for what it was, but ultimately, upon reflection, he was protecting himself because I was not ready to admit to him, or anybody else, that I was gay. It seems that he knew me better than I knew myself.

Losing this friend, I believe, is what triggered a crisis. When I was around 40 years old, I spiralled into what some might call a midlife crisis. I barely spoke and I withdrew from everyone close to me. My wife was worried and spoke to other people about how concerned she was. We finally decided that I needed to do something about it, so I made an appointment to see a doctor. After an examination and a short chat, I was declared clinically depressed and signed papers to register myself as such. Medication was prescribed for my depression, and I was informed that I would not see results for a few weeks. Deep down I knew there was something more to this, but I couldn't quite put my finger on it. I took the pills for about a week and they calmed me down enough to sort my thoughts out. Then the white noise abated. Not long after that, I woke up one morning and was sitting on the edge of the bed. I looked in the mirror and admitted to myself for the first time in my life that I'm gay. I immediately threw the pills down the toilet, took a deep breath and braced myself for what was to come! My life was about to change forever.

Coming out

Around 15 years after I married my best friend, I found the courage to come out. That was some time ago now. A lot changed gradually over the first two months, and then rapidly over the next six or so years. Perhaps I was naïve, but I thought the best way forward was to be totally honest with my best friend. This was a huge mistake! The fall out was chaotic and disappointing in both the way people would react and how decisions were to be made. My 'ideal' family life was to be torn from me very quickly.

We had three beautiful children who were still fairly young at the time I came out. I had a high-level position in the Catholic education system, a wonderful home and enjoyed everything a beachside lifestyle, in Western Australia could offer. We were considered a close-knit family and were good friends with families similar to ours. I instilled in my children attributes such as honesty, care for others, and responsibility. I had a motto that I went by, 'There's no such thing as a problem you can't solve together as a family.' We would often talk about our day and refer to this motto regularly as we solved issues such as bullying at school or ways around being swamped by too many tasks at work. It was this motto, in particular, that would drive me to come out to my family as soon as I could.

I was 40 years old when I came out and fully acknowledge that I didn't have a tortured life. It was quite easy going, but everything began to change. The last 12 months before I came out were horrendous for me, as my health deteriorated and my mind became more confused. I couldn't deny my feelings any longer and I needed to accept the fact that I was gay. I had ignored any idea or signs of being gay, as I had certain expectations of living a traditional life in a straight world.

I needed to speak to someone about how I was feeling and the only place I could find at that time was the West Australian AIDS Council. I felt I needed to speak to a counsellor about being gay now that I had accepted it, and to assist me with the next steps. I sought this support before I came out to anyone else, almost as a way of seeking a second opinion in case I was wrong!

After a few sessions with the counsellor, I announced to him that I was going to tell my wife. The counsellor thought I should hold off and not rush into it, but that was now not possible for me. I believed with all my heart that 'there was no such thing as a problem you can't solve together as a family', so here was a chance to test that out. Initially, my wife was shocked, of course, but took the news surprisingly well. For the next couple of months, we appeared to stay good friends. It got to the point that we were talking about how life could be and how we wanted it to be. Together, we talked to the children and talked about some of the changes that were going to take place but stressed the importance of working through this as a family. The appearance that this could work was short lived.

Our relationship soured quickly, when outside influences began to 'coach' my wife in an effort to get the best for her out of this 'new situation'. This became obvious one day when my wife asked me to pick the kids up after a day at the beach. Upon arriving home, I discovered the locks on the doors had been changed and a male friend of my wife's was sitting in his car parked across the street. This was the moment my life changed, and all I could do was to take advice from my young daughter who called out to me, 'Dad, just leave it and let's go.' We did leave, but my heart stayed. Later that night, I returned the children back to their home, leaving them at the front door, and I was never to set foot in that home, my home, ever again!

Obviously, having been kicked out of my home, I had to find somewhere else to live. The naïve part of me did not set up a new bank account or put money aside before coming out, so the next few years were going to be tough, financially and emotionally. The hardest part was watching, mostly from the sideline, how my decision had fall out for my children. For me, they were the ones to be protected. They had to be, because it wasn't their fault and they were too young to care for themselves. Unfortunately, my wife didn't share these thoughts, often citing the idea, that she needed to heal herself before she could help anyone else. Lack of funds restricted my accommodation choices and the possibility of enough rooms for the children became impossible. My first apartment was a small studio around 30 square metres, and I had to be financially assisted by my mother to pay the bond. I would consider that a definite low point in my life.

For a while, the rest of my family did not know that I had come out. I decided to fly to Melbourne because I wanted to tell my mum in person. By now my dad had passed away. Mum's first reaction was quizzical, asking, 'That's a bit weird, isn't it?' Immediately something must have changed on my face because to her credit, she went on to say, with a hint of regret in her voice, 'I've said the wrong thing, haven't I?'. My sister was there as always and her reaction was clear- she was okay with it and she had my back. We went on to have a really good conversation about everything. My dear mum now defends me and my community if she hears anyone putting us down. She often tells me that someone had said something and she put them straight (pardon the pun!). My mother is about to turn 90 years old – definitely ahead of her time!

I have no regrets. I have three amazing children who love me for who I am, and I will always be there for them. If anyone got me through the very difficult days, it was them. A hug and a smile from them will always brighten my day.

Life after coming out

After coming out, I became very introspective as many people were asking me questions, and I had to think deeply about my answers. For example, why didn't I know this about myself before and start to question a lot of things? I remembered things that I now see as signs that I was gay, but I wondered why I didn't notice it at the time. The only explanation that I can offer, is that I did not want to be gay. I wasn't hiding anything from anyone, although perhaps I was. I was flat out denying that it was possible. I did not fit the gay stereotypes and narrative I was fed as a kid, so therefore I did not think I was gay. Perhaps as I get on in years, I will have a better explanation, but for now I just breathe and accept where I am.

Some people just know they are gay and tell everybody, or they move away and begin a different life. This wasn't going to be easy for me, I knew it, but it was going to test my resilience and character many times over. I was going to survive this and be the best damn gay-dad possible for my kids! I knew I would be okay in the end, and although there were times, I was so low, that I considered taking my life, a photo of my kids kept me going. I just needed to prove to them that even when life is hard, there are still things that can keep you smiling. I hope the truth is, they do not actually know how hard life was for me, but no doubt, as they grow up, they will want to discuss things or perhaps things will pop up unexpectedly in conversation. We will address them when the time is right.

I am definitely more focused now on priorities and what is more important to me, rather than on how people viewed me before I came out. In the past, material things were important to me, including a job with prestige, lovely cars and vacations. This changed once I came out, as I realised my emotional happiness was worth more to me than accumulated wealth. I no longer have the trappings of keeping up appearances as my life is now simpler and much more fun!

The most stress I've experienced since coming out would be my divorce and everything associated with that, especially the impact on my children. It was a negative experience for everyone, but at least there was an end date. Divorce is never easy on anyone and especially the fallout for kids. If you are reading this and are going through a divorce, and you have children, please put them first. Always put them first!

I do miss the family times and the closeness I had with my kids. I often reminisce about watching TV with the kids on the sofa. We were always a pile of people, laying over each other, intertwined and close as we laughed through our favourite shows. It is this closeness, the times we laughed out loud, or the quiet times just before bedtime that I miss the most. Once the locks on the door were changed, those opportunities were taken away and replaced with shorter opportunities when the children would come to my apartment for dinner or we would eat together at our favourite restaurant. Even school graduations and birthday celebrations would need to have separate events because of the feelings my coming out caused for my wife. Unfortunately, those feelings have not subsided, although time has marched on so significantly.

My friendships changed also. Before I came out, we regularly socialised with four other families. They were very good friends and we had 12 children amongst us who all loved playing together. The other husbands and I were really close mates, and often we would have coffee together or hit the pubs to share beers. I considered them to be my brothers and trusted them completely. I would have sought their counsel when I had come to terms with my coming out, but I never got the chance to come out to them. I discovered that during the months when my wife and I were appearing to be friends, she was visiting all our friends and neighbours telling them that I was gay. In terms of coming out, you could say I really only came out to four people

– my wife and three children. She outed me to everyone else! Coming out to my friends was not so much a celebration, but a need to explain myself to people that were both shocked and upset after hearing stories from my wife. One close friend, in particular, became quite angry with me. Being a strict Catholic, he couldn't come to terms with my news. The other families couldn't deal with the issues surrounding the fall out. Often, they say they were targeted because they had spent time with me and therefore had to protect themselves from homophobic abuse. I haven't seen them since.

As mentioned earlier, I worked in the Catholic education system, and of course, their doctrine is that it is not acceptable to be gay. I did have a clause in my work contract along the lines of – I had to live in accordance to the teachings of the church. My contract was due to be renewed as a team leader. At the time I had a senior position within the Catholic education system. Although not talked about, it was probably known that I was gay as I had been out for five to six years. My wife was also teaching in the Catholic system and made it known that we had divorced because I was gay. This reliable source of information was acknowledged many times when I was encouraged by a number of people to go to the Director and tell him that the rumours were false.

It was after I married my husband in Sweden that the uproar started. A group of people from the community continually complained to the Catholic hierarchy about my marriage and they wanted action taken against me. It was a situation they felt they needed to deal with. As a result, I lost my job and once again things looked grim. Luckily, I picked up another position and being married helped me cope with the fallout. The saying 'don't ask, don't tell' is standard practice in Catholic circles, but the experience of leaving that culture and be free to tell my story was like a heavy weight being lifted from my shoulders.

I thought I was really happy in my past life, and I thought I knew what love was, but now I know what love is and experience it daily in the relationship I have with my husband. Part of that is because I am now living a more truthful life, and I am who I want to be. I believe I am a better father now that I'm more authentic, and my children can really see me for who I am. The best times are when my children, husband and I get together. We are a different family group than we once were, but one to be cherished all the same.

Influences in search of happiness

I have come to understand that my husband is my soulmate, as corny as it sounds. I feel privileged that I have found someone who has helped me understand who I am by being patient and forgiving as I searched for myself. If we had met earlier it probably wouldn't have worked, mostly because I was yet to admit to myself that I was gay. When we met, I had been through most of the messy part of my coming out story and things were beginning to settle down. We met in Sweden in January 2012, when I was speaking at a conference in Malmö. It was a chance meeting that had a significant effect on changing our lives forever and for the better. For a number of years, we travelled across the world to see each other, clocking up the flight hours to incredible heights. I think the longest we were apart was around four months. He came to live in Australia for a couple of years and now we live in Sweden.

My eldest sister was very influential for my happiness. She didn't miss a beat when I told her. She supported me through my divorce and made it very clear that my being gay didn't matter one bit. At the end of the day, she wanted me to be happy and our relationship has continued to grow stronger. She and her husband are two people that I know I can, and will, rely on no matter what's happening in my life. We always have a wonderful time when we get together with them.

I feel blessed that I got a chance to enhance my life. It was great before, but now it's even better. It seems the best things from my earlier life have stayed with me, and I have had the chance to add more 'best things'. I feel like I've given myself a second chance to live an amazing life and I'm not going to take it for granted. I literally had to fight hard and sacrificed much to get this far.

Biggest challenges in life

Was it worth coming out? Yes, it absolutely was, although at times I wondered if I had done the wrong thing. When my kids were upset, and wanted things to go back to 'normal', I pondered the idea that it was a mistake. It was only when I thought about things logically, that it made sense to keep going and make it worthwhile. I just could not live with myself if I caused all this chaos for nothing, just to give up or not make a go of it. Now, I sometimes think about my life, and what it would be like if I had come out earlier, but of course I wouldn't want that. I couldn't imagine life without my kids, so the timing was right.

Once everything was out in the open, I had to, of course, move out of the family home. I remember returning home one day to pick up my personal belongings, only to find them literally thrown out onto the driveway in a pile. That hurt, and no doubt the action was designed to do that. I picked up what I could, in the time I had and went on my way. I also lost my job, lost my friends, and couldn't see the kids very often. It was difficult moving from a large family home to living in a tiny apartment. These were big challenges for me.

Seeing the children was one of the biggest challenges, but at the same time, the most rewarding. It was, and continues to be, important for me that they know I am there, and that I love them. Many times, I found them upset, on the side of the road when they were dropped off by their mother. Her refusal to walk them to the door or discuss their needs with me was painfully hard to deal with. I remember one night: it was raining and cold outside. I was down on a busy street, having been told that she was dropping my son off to me, five minutes before she arrived. I went to meet her at the agreed meeting place, but she had arrived some moments before I got there. As she sped off, not wanting to talk to me, I could make out a lonely figure in the rain. Here was my youngest boy, not yet 10 years old, standing in the rain, holding his bag. There were many situations like that, and they were difficult for me to understand and process.

I have one brother who, for some reason, could not accept me being gay. I suspect there are reasons, but we don't speak. He, and his family have not invited me to any family events that they have organised, and I have been told that he keeps up the stereotyped conversations that I heard throughout my childhood. It is a challenge, but time and distance has helped put it where it belongs – in the past. I remember being at a family wedding shortly after I came out. It was an informal affair with guests standing around in the garden as the ceremony took place. He stood behind me, quietly offering disparaging comments about my lifestyle choices, and sniggering at lame jokes he told anyone standing close to him. I can't lie, it definitely hurt at the time, but I've moved on. He has his own demons to deal with.

But perhaps the biggest challenge in life, after coming out was the fact that it was 'assumed' I was alright. I had been kicked out of my family home, lost my job, lost full time access to my children and had little money given I was paying child support, divorce lawyers and bank loans on top of newly acquired rent and living demands. To me, it seemed that because I had 'chosen' this way forward, I must have been happy with the outcome, that I was coping just fine and there was no need to check in. That was a bitter pill to swallow. Only two family members would ring to ask how I was – my sister and my mother. It wasn't that I was looking for sympathy, it was just that most people treated it as if it was a planned track in my life, a sensational alternative to what I had before, when in reality it was far from that. Coming out is a very hard decision to make. When someone comes out to you, be there for them, not just the day after or the moment they tell you, but check in regularly, because like any major decision you make in life, there are days you are glad you made the decision, but an equal number of days, if not more, when you regret it.

What would you tell your younger self?

The pain of coming out is not greater than the pain of staying in. I can only imagine what life would be like now if I hadn't come out. Physically, logically, I can imagine my old life, but not emotionally. I get a glimpse of 'straight life' every time I turn on the television or visit my family. It's easy to imagine myself in the shoes of a straight man – I walked in them for such a long time. Emotionally, though, I can't. I am not sure how I would have been able to keep it all together. Living a double life, or a life where I denied my true feelings would have eventually led to a breakdown or worse.

Being honest with yourself is very empowering. I got sick and tired of pretending to be straight and trying to act and live like a straight man – it was exhausting, and as I have described previously, harmful to my body and mind. It does take courage to admit something to yourself that you are something you don't want to be, but once across the threshold of realisation, you are more powerful than you ever thought possible. I am a better person, father, husband, brother and friend than I ever thought possible. I am finally calm.

People will understand you coming out and then choose their behaviour. You can help them understand but you can't influence their reaction. Some will accept you the way you are and some will not – try not to take it personally as it is not so much about you as it is to do with their own struggles.

Ultimately, living up to other people's standards and expectations is not what life is about. It's about reaching your goals and participating in society and life without the restrictions of behaving in a certain way. Now I can live my life much more fully as I'm not scared of being judged by anyone, anymore. I can accept that people are not happy with my way of life, and will judge me, but I'm okay with that. Each to their own!

I do ponder sometimes why I hadn't come out any earlier and what would life be like now. However, I don't dwell on that too often. If I didn't come out at the right time, I wouldn't have my beautiful children and may not have met my wonderful husband. We have to learn from our experiences, move on and make peace with what has happened in the past. I think being part of the process of telling my story is part of the way forward.

Greg

The younger years

My childhood was spent running around the area of Parkdale, Victoria where I lived with my parents, older brother, David, older sister, Dianne, and younger sister, Rosemary. I would describe my family by saying that we make the Royal Family look like the Brady Bunch – highly dysfunctional! I attended Parkdale Primary School then Parkdale High School. My mum was a rather blunt person and she insisted when I was in my teen years that I join the local Cubs then Sea Scouts, judo (I hated that) and gymnastics. I asked her one day, why I had to do these things. Her reply was, 'Because your brother's an arsehole and you're not going to turn out the same.' Obviously, I was much more obliging than my brother, David, and did not aspire to be like him. My dad was quietly dignified and unassuming. My younger sister, Rosemary, was unfortunately known for her repeated suicide attempts. My dear dad, who was a man of few words, after one of the many threats of suicide from Rosemary, said one day, 'Well, I hope next time she gets it right!' That would now be about 32 years ago, and Rosemary is still alive and kicking. Her struggles with alcohol have not abated and David has faced a similar battle. I, fortunately, am now the opposite and don't drink at all.

Generally, my childhood was happy with not too many cares in the world. My happiest memories as a kid were playing in the local tip which is now the Walter Galt Reserve in Parkdale, riding my bike with friends and playing in the Mordialloc Creek. All quite normal stuff for kids of that era. As long as I was home by sunset, I was free to roam wherever I wanted.

One day, when I was 15, I was sitting at the kitchen table reading the *Truth* newspaper. My favourite section was called 'Heart Balm', which was the equivalent of a 'Dear Abby' column. I found it quite fascinating reading about people's problems. There was an article in there about homosexuals, and I asked my mum what a homosexual was. She said it was a man that would prefer to love a man rather than a woman. I asked her if that was bad, and I can't remember her exact reply, but I do remember she didn't imply that it was either. I also noticed that any stories of homosexual people in the newspaper were located on the pages that had sordid stories about deviates. These were different times compared to now. People's lifestyles were scrutinised and judged. I remember my dad inviting a friend home from his work one day. Whenever Mum and Dad talked about him, it was in hushed tones because he had been divorced, and that was frowned upon. Even though the critical judgement was not openly discussed, the hushed tones were enough to signify that something was wrong, making it a bad thing.

The realisation

When I was about 18 years old, I was shopping with Mum at Southland Shopping Centre when I spotted a good-looking man with blond hair. All he was doing was rummaging through clothes in a shop, and I couldn't stop looking at him and felt besotted by him. That was the first time I had an inkling that I was attracted to men, but it would be a few years later before I acted on anything. At 21, I had a girlfriend for five minutes; I tried it and didn't like it! Up until this time in my life, I thought I was the only one who felt this way about other men, as I had never been exposed to homosexuality.

There was another newspaper called the *Melbourne Star Observer* that was specifically published for the gay community. In it there was an article that listed all the gay venues in Melbourne at that time. I was keen to find out what they were like as I didn't even know places like this existed. I had finally come home. I could now go out to party and look at other guys without the fear of being attacked or ridiculed. It was a safe place. My favourite venue was called Mandate located in Carlisle Street, St Kilda. This is where I found my community and best friend Michael. He was keen to have a relationship with me, but I wasn't interested in him that way. I was now firmly ensconced in the gay lifestyle but didn't come out for another five years.

Coming out

When I was in my mid-twenties, I was sitting in my sister, Dianne's, kitchen and decided to tell her I was gay. Up until this time, no one in my family knew. When I told her, she said, 'It doesn't matter, I still love you.' I felt such relief, as it helped me to not feel so disgusted with myself if she could still love me.

When I was 40 years old, my parents by then had left Parkdale and had been living in Echuca for seven years after Dad's retirement. I received a call from Mum to tell me Dad had passed away after a second stroke. His funeral was held in Melbourne, so Mum came down and stayed with me for two weeks. On one of these days after the funeral, I was sitting with Mum and she said, 'I need something to think about rather than your father', I then promptly replied with, 'Oh, by the way, I'm gay and I'm HIV positive.' I certainly gave her something else to think about, probably not what she was expecting, but she seemed to take it in her stride. It looks like I may have inherited Mum's bluntness!

It's funny, but even though I never told my dad I was gay, when he was in hospital after his first stroke, he would make comments to me like, 'Oh look, there's a handsome young doctor.' I think it was his way of saying it's okay without having to talk about it – bless! He really was a gentle soul.

Life after coming out

As my coming out stories are not overly dramatic, and there was no massive build up or negative feedback after coming out; life went on as normal.

When I was 42 years old, I met Mark from Tasmania at the Exchange Hotel in Prahran. We became friends which then lead to a long-term relationship of seven years. In the end, I realised I wanted more from life as he was happy to live like a boring married couple, whereas I still wanted to go out and enjoy life.

This was brought to light when we had travelled to Sydney for Mardi Gras, and upon our arrival he was quite content to stay in the hotel and watch television rather than go out and have some fun. That was the beginning of the end; we only lasted another couple of years together. Other than that relationship, I've been on my own and content with my own company.

Influences in search of happiness

I made reference earlier to finding my community. This consisted of friends I made at Mandate where we became a very close-knit bunch – Michael, Joan and Steph. We became a 'framily', a cross between family and friends. We were always together and they accepted me for who I am. I could tell them anything and they wouldn't bat an eyelid. To this day, we are still lifelong friends.

Biggest challenges in life

At the age of 26, I moved out of home into a one-bedroom apartment which was the same year I came out. It was the year of 'outs' for me. At this time of my life, I didn't like being gay or like who I was. A consequence of this, was drinking way too much on my own at home to dull the disgust inside of me. Then something happened that changed my life. A little girl, six years old, named Kylie Maybury, was murdered by a family friend of hers. She was raped and left to die on the side of the road in Coburg. I knew her and her mother, and it was hard to get my head around this horrific crime. I sat there one day and asked myself some questions in my head. Firstly, whether I could do that to a child, and the answer to that was 'never'. Then I asked myself whether I could do that to a partner, and the answer was 'never'. I continued through different scenarios and always came up with the same answer: 'never'. This was the moment I realised I was not a horrible person and the disgust I had for myself slowly began to dissipate, and I started to like who I was, and life seemed much lighter than before. It was a simple process, but it worked for me.

It was now 1994 and I had turned 40. It was also the year my dad passed away and I contracted HIV. Let's just say it was not one of my best years. I still don't know who I got it from. I decided to randomly get tested one day for STDs not thinking at all that I had HIV as I had no symptoms. What was really weird was one of the directives from the doctor. He told me to eat cake! I walked away wondering what he meant. I can only surmise that he meant for me to put weight on to fight the disease as the people who died from AIDS were reduced to skin and bone. The first lot of drugs I was on made me feel sick, making it a common occurrence for me to throw up on the way to work in someone's garden. I was on that medication for about three years. As time went on, new improved drugs were discovered with less side effects, however, it did affect the muscle mass in my legs making it harder to walk and I tired easily. As the side effects were fairly significant, I was told by my doctor to have a 'drug holiday'. This was a time to give my body a break for two years from the poisonous medication that was keeping the HIV at bay. When I was first diagnosed, I would swallow up to 10 tablets per day, now I'm down to one tablet per day with few side effects – thank goodness for continued research.

In the early to mid-eighties, I have vivid memories of opening the Obituaries in the *Melbourne Star Observer*, seeing page after page of those who had passed away from AIDS. Many times, I saw names of people I recognised or friends of friends. Somehow,

I managed to avoid the Grim Reaper as I contracted HIV when it was no longer a death sentence. If you want, you can search on YouTube for the Grim Reaper advertisements if you don't know what they are. Horrifying times!

What would you tell your younger self?

I would tell my younger self that everything will turn out okay. Once I realised that I wasn't such a bad person after all, I became a happier human being. I stopped judging myself so harshly. This helped free me up to enjoy all that life had to offer, because no longer did I care what other people thought of me. Try it, it's absolutely liberating!

James

The younger years

I'm now a permanent resident of Australia, but I grew up in Berkshire, UK, with one brother, Tony. My parents divorced when I was nine years old then remarried about four years later. I suppose they realised the grass wasn't greener on the other side. My childhood was what I would call 'normal' for a working-class family. My parents worked hard to give us a good life, and a big part of my life was competition show jumping horses. There was the odd comment from people about my sport being gay, but it never seemed to affect me. Interestingly, if I had belonged to a wealthy family where I attended a private school, my choice of sport would have been more accepted for a male. My brother and I had totally different interests as Tony was quite the lad who loved football and sports that were rough – I did not. Whilst living in Berkshire, I never met a lesbian or a gay guy, so I was not exposed to an alternative way of life.

Having said that, I was not exposed to homophobia either, but the expectation was to live a traditional lifestyle with a wife and children in a nice house.

Throughout my teens I had crushes on various girls but never dated anyone. The boys didn't catch my eye at all through my teens, as in my head, I always thought I was straight. I didn't start dating until my early twenties, with the longest relationship I had was about one year. I went on many dates with girls in the hope of finding the right one to create a family with. Friends would organise blind dates for me, but I constantly made an excuse that there was no spark. In my mind, I honestly believed I was not gay. I never felt like I was deceiving anyone; I would just tell myself that I hadn't found the right person.

In my late twenties, while quite drunk, I started messing around with a guy I met online and one thing led to another. I justified my behaviour by thinking that I was bisexual so there was no need to explain my behaviour to anyone, plus, I wasn't interested in having a relationship with him, as for me, it was purely physical. My dream of the traditional family was still alive and well.

At the age of 34, I decided to move to Australia. When visiting my brother, Tony, who was now living in Melbourne, I witnessed a lifestyle that I wanted to be a part of. I was also at a crossroads in my career, so the idea of new career opportunities and living in a warmer climate was quite appealing to me. At this stage I was still going on dates with girls, as boys were not part of the equation yet.

The realisation

For many years, I honestly thought I was bisexual and only hooked up with men in private for physical connection, not envisaging any emotional connection or future with a man. At around 36 years of age, I met a guy called Andy who asked me out for a drink at a bar. My initial thought was about where we're going to meet, as it meant going out in public, but he suggested meeting near my work and I felt comfortable enough with that. Up until then, I was living in the dark depths of the closet. I had an instant connection with Andy, which threw me as I had made a decision to not get emotionally involved with a man, as I had not yet accepted the fact that I was gay. The game had now changed. After that meeting at the bar with Andy, we were in constant contact and began dating. I was now at another crossroads: do I continue to live a lie or face up to my new reality?

After a short time of dating Andy, I knew I had to confess to him that I was not out yet. I rang him one day when I was at work and told him that I was not out of the closet and that I actually lived in Coogee. I had told him I lived in Clovelly, as I didn't want to meet him near my home in case anyone saw us. Looking back, it seems so ridiculous now. Andy took if very well, I even gave him an 'out' if he wanted, but he stuck with me and became a wonderful support for me as I emerged into the world as a gay man.

Coming out

The first person I made my announcement to was a female work colleague I felt very comfortable with, as I knew she had many gay friends. I suggested we go for a coffee and a chat. I found myself unable to get my words out and then I had broken down as I was so emotional. My poor friend thought I was terminally ill as I was so distraught and tongue-tied. I was finally able to say I was dating – and they were a guy. She was so happy for me and burst into tears herself. I felt like I was on cloud nine, it was so amazing! After that I began to tell selected friends, but I noticed I would tell them by saying I was dating a guy rather than saying I was gay. There was still a small part of me that worried about what people would think, and using those words seemed to make it more comfortable for myself, even though the outcome is the same. I still hadn't told my family.

It took me approximately six months after first telling my friends that I was gay, and I couldn't hold off any longer telling my family. My younger brother, Tony, was still living in Melbourne and my parents still lived in the UK. I flew down from Sydney to visit Tony and his partner, Nicola, to tell them the news. They didn't know I was coming down to make any announcement, but they thought something was up when they saw me throwing back the drinks for Dutch courage. For some stupid reason I thought Tony might not be okay with this news, and I worried that he may not accept me. It may have had something to do with him being so blokey and not knowing anyone who was gay, but deep down I knew that he would be accepting. Unfortunately, the unreasonable voices in my head were louder than the voice of reason. Once I plucked up the courage to tell them, Tony became teary and emotional while Nicola jumped up and hugged me. Tony was upset thinking that I had been suffering for years by being in the closet and that he wasn't there to help me. I assured him that wasn't the case as I didn't feel like I suffered that much. I had the canny knack of being able to compartmentalise my life. This worked just fine until I couldn't ignore my attraction to men bubbling to the surface. I would justify my hooking up with guys by telling myself I was just experimenting, and it was successful until I met Andy and feelings were involved.

The next and final step in coming out to those I love, was telling my parents in the UK. This had to be done over the phone which I found a bit easier than face to face. Once the chit chat with Mum was out of the way, I again became quite emotional as I told her that I was dating a guy. Her reply was, 'That's okay, I used to work with a guy who was gay.' I think that was her way of saying it's all good. She then started to ask me questions about Andy and making sure I was okay emotionally. After the phone call was over, I received a message from my dad as Mum had told him my news. He texted me to say that all is good, don't worry and that he was proud of me. That was my last hurdle that I jumped with a positive outcome.

Life after coming out

Officially, I only came out four years ago when I was 37 years old. As I was in a relationship when I came out and in a happy place, I had this feeling of freedom that I never really experienced before. Being in love with a man was new to me so I just felt happiness. With Andy by my side, I almost felt fearless as if nothing could hurt me, as if he was my armour against any negativity. Having said that, none really came my way. I didn't actually feel suppressed before I came out, so the only change to my life was that I was dating a guy rather than a girl, so life essentially went on as normal.

Influences in search of happiness

My current partner, Chris, would probably be my biggest influence on my happiness. I reached a point in my life where I was keen to settle down even though I was content with myself, I wanted someone to share my life with. The dating scene was great fun, but at the same time very frustrating. For example, I would be talking to a guy via an app for a few days, and then he'd casually drop in the conversation that he was in a relationship, but it's okay as it's an open relationship. This is quite common amongst the gay community; however, it was not what I wanted.

Like anyone trying to find a partner, you have to kiss a few frogs, but I'd kissed so many that I was losing faith in finding anyone I could connect with on all levels. My faith was restored when I met Chris as I have finally found my partner in crime. We just clicked and fortunately want the same things in life, of which one of those is creating our own family together. So, my vision of having a family one day is now more a reality than it's ever been before.

Biggest challenges in life

When my relationship with Andy ended after about a year together, I was left feeling lonely and isolated in a gay world as all my friends were straight, making it difficult to discuss my broken heart. I then decided that I needed to break out and begin dating and making friends that were gay. As time went on, I began to create new friendship groups of people who understood me with no explanations required.

One of my biggest challenges was accepting that I was gay, as I believed I would have to give up my dream of having a family or traditional lifestyle, as that is all I ever wanted. I can see now that I had a preconception of what a gay life entailed. For me, I thought it was more about being single, partying and sleeping around even if you're in a relationship. The more I emersed myself in the gay world, the more I realised this was not the case. Yes, my preconceptions were true, but I made the mistake of applying this to all gay men rather than a small percentage. I have no problem with people living a hedonistic lifestyle, and I did do this for a while after I came out, but it wasn't a lifestyle that I wanted to maintain. Because I came out at such a late age, for me it was the equivalent of adolescent behaviour before settling down. I needed to experience being single, gay and partying for fun. I was like a kid in a candy shop.

What would you tell your younger self?

Surround yourself with family and friends whose goal it is to love and support you no matter what. I would encourage fearlessness so that you can live the life you want to live by being true to yourself.

Even if you can only be brave enough to speak to one person you trust about how you feel or how you are confused and don't know what to do. That person could give you advice that could make the difference between living a happy or an unhappy life.

Dale

The younger years

My early childhood years were spent in an idyllic part of country Victoria called Tongala located near Echuca. I have three siblings, an older brother, Noel, and two younger sisters, Lorelle and Carolann, and my parents are still together. Dad was an interstate truck driver and Mum stayed home to look after us kids. Life was fairly adventurous growing up in the country as there were plenty of places to play and get up to mischief. I remember our household being fairly drama free. The biggest challenge was dodging the tiger snakes that frequented the backyard and surrounding bushlands!

When I was seven years old, the family uprooted and moved to the big smoke in Sydney to a suburb called Five Dock. Three years later, at the age of 10, we moved to Toongabbie in New South Wales where I attended Grantham High School until Year 10. I did get picked on at high school as I was a little runt and a country boy. I must have still had a bit of country mentality in me. Fortunately, I found some good friends at school and as we all enjoyed singing, we became a very close group. Even though I was called a 'poofter', it seemed not to stick or phase me that much. Keeping in mind that in the early seventies being gay was still illegal, so I was the trifecta – gay, illegal and underage!

When I was 16 years old, I left school to begin working at a radiator company in the office doing admin work and smoking like a chimney (it was legal to smoke in the office in those days). I procured this job through my older brother as he worked on the floor as a foreman. The job only lasted a few months as I was too busy socialising and, too often, not turning up for work. Not a great start to a career but moving on gave me the opportunity to work in retail and hospitality to which I was much more suited, and that's where I stayed for most of my working life.

The realisation

When I was four years old in Tongala, I have a vivid memory of a little glass house (used as a hot house to grow plants) that was next to the main house. I used to steal Mum's stockings and hide them in the glass house to try them on later. Everyone played doctors and nurses growing up, but I played doctors and doctors not connecting that was possibly my preference.

When going through puberty the penny began to drop. I'd been sneaking out to gay nightclubs in Sydney since I was 14 years old. I started with ballroom dancing classes, that was on the up and up, then I progressed to gay nightclubs in the evening at Oxford Street. Being gay evolved quite naturally for me as I'd always been quite comfortable in my own skin. I can see now that I'm one of the fortunate ones that didn't fight how I naturally felt – I was able to embrace my lifestyle with gusto!

Coming out

I made the decision at 15 years old to come out to my mum. I had been pretending to go to ballroom dancing lessons but really going to nightclubs drinking for the past 18 months, so I felt it was time to come out. It was Queen's Birthday weekend and I had been invited to spend it with a group of gay friends. I told Mum that I was staying at a school friend's place for the three-day weekend. On the Sunday, my drinking friends dropped me near home as we were having a BBQ, and I needed to pick up some meat from home to have at the BBQ. Mum saw me run back to the car which was in the opposite direction to my school friends place that I was meant to be staying at. Rookie error if you're trying to cover your tracks. On the Monday night my friends and I went to a nightclub, even though I knew I had school the next day. While at the nightclub, I made the decision to get really drunk and tell my mum that I was gay. I finally boarded the train to go home at 2 am on the Tuesday morning. By this time, I was in tears as I walked up the garden path to my front door. I knew Mum was waiting for me, as I had seen the curtain fall back across the window as I approached the house. She had been searching for me at my friend's place where I was meant to be. No mobiles in those days!

So, I walked in the door, drunk and crying and promptly announced to Mum that I was gay, to which she replied, 'I already know that and you're still going to school tomorrow!' She was more furious that I was drunk than being gay. It was a very long school day! That morning though, before I went to school, I had a quick discussion with Mum in her bedroom. She confirmed that the family still love me, but said, 'Don't flaunt the fact that you're gay.' So that was that.

Coming out gave me the courage to be myself and more resilient as no one could hurt me now that my family knew I was gay. There were no more secrets as there was nothing left to hide. To this day I've not had a discussion with my dad about being gay. When I turned 16, I was going out one night and my dad said, 'If you go out that door, don't come back!' I think he didn't want me hanging around with gay people but didn't actually say those words. We were both very stubborn, so when I was at the nightclub that night after walking out the door, I cried all night to my friends, knowing I couldn't go back home. In the morning I came across a newspaper that was advertising a boarding house. I then went home, packed my things and Mum gave me some money to help me with the cost of moving out. Fortunately, at that time I was working at the radiator company, so I at least I had an income.

Life after coming out

After I came out, I definitely felt more secure within myself and I noticed that I had gained confidence and stood up for myself more. Between the ages of 16 and 18 I began performing in shows at the Tropicana Club in Oxford Street, Sydney. We did drag shows and production numbers and I absolutely loved it! I then moved to Melbourne for about three to four years where I go-go danced in a cage at the Key Club in Carlton. Because it was illegal to be gay, you literally had to have a key to get into the Key Club to get through to reception. This was a nightclub for gay men where we could be ourselves without being judged, and we looked out for each other.

Most of my working life has been spent in the Arts arena where I've met all types of people in the entertaining industry. I believe that if I hadn't come out, I wouldn't have had all the fabulous experiences and met all the colourful people in my life.

My family and extended family members were fine with me being gay, except for one uncle who, unfortunately, happened to be my favourite uncle. Once he found out I was gay, he even stopped me babysitting my younger cousins. I also feel sad that I was not able to have a full relationship with my aunty, due to my uncle's homophobia that was fuelled by his Catholic beliefs. My thoughts on religion now, are that I'm quite comfortable with anyone practicing a religion, as long as they don't hurt others in the name of religion or try to shove it down my throat. I believe everyone has the right to their opinions, as do I, but I don't tolerate fanaticism.

When I was 28 years old, my parents decided to renew their vows and the celebration was at Pizza Hut. I wasn't happy with the red and white checked table clothes, so my partner at the time, Malcolm, and I, decided to spruce up the Pizza Hut with white table clothes, pearl balloons on the chairs, white candles on all the tables and a homemade wedding cake. Mum and Dad didn't have much money and we wanted to make it a special occasion. Before we left for the function, we had to have the obligatory family photos. Dad announced that he wanted to have a photo with his boys. My brother and I wandered over to have our photo taken and Dad said, 'I want Malcolm as well, he's like a son to me.' My chest absolutely exploded with joy and it was in that moment that I knew he had accepted me and us as a couple.

Influences in search of happiness

For whatever reason, I was always able to stand up for myself against bullies and people who targeted me because I was gay. Once I came out, there was no reason to hide anymore and I didn't care who knew. This meant no one could hold anything over me. So, I could live the life I wanted to live. I remember an incident in secondary school when I was around 16 years. There was one boy in particular who liked to bully me about being gay. One day, he pushed my head into the door jam and was calling me gay. I turned around and said in a really loud voice, 'Go and hit me anyway, as you'll call me a liar no matter what I say!' I waited for the punch, but he didn't hit me as another guy stepped in and told him to leave me alone. I'd had an absolute gutful of this treatment and now that my family knew I was gay, all my fears had disappeared and I had nothing to lose. Once I announced that, the other kids began saying, 'Leave him alone, he's okay,' and from then on, he didn't bother me again. He couldn't be the big man he was trying to be, and he knew he couldn't hurt me anymore with his accusations.

I feel that there's no one person that's influenced me in a positive way as I've been able to organically see the brighter side of life, and I have some sort of built-in resilience. Having said that, my grandparents on my mother's side were quite influential in my life. They were very protective of me and instilled in me that all will be okay, so maybe that has helped me be strong and resilient in the face of adversity.

Performing has always been a big part of my life and glamour drag is my passion. I dress up as a woman and perform a dance sequence while lip syncing. I love the costumes, putting on my own makeup and I'm transported to another world. Many of my friends that I performed with are now transgender. When I was 18, I went to a transgender psychologist (my grandmother took me, bless her) to explore the feelings I had, but I realised I didn't want to transition as I was able to fulfill my yearning as a female by dressing in drag. I now label what I do as performance art, and I'm content with that as I identify as a man who happens to have feminine traits.

I'm currently very happy in my life whether I'm in a relationship or not. I've learnt to love my own company as well as love myself. Even though it's corny to say, but if I died tomorrow, I would die happy!

Biggest challenges in life

In my life, I have been raped three times at the age of 15, 24 and 47 years old. Without going into detail, I want to say that 'no means no'! So, if someone physically holds you down against your will and you're saying 'no', then it's rape. When I was 15, as it was illegal to be gay, I couldn't even go to the Police. If you are ever in this situation, please report the abuse. The way I cope with this violation is by seeing it as an abuse of my body, not my mind. By framing it in this way, it helps me to not see myself as a victim because it wasn't my fault and it wasn't a personal attack; I just happened to be the person they chose.

About 10 years ago, I had a massive lifestyle change, as I had to stop drinking after my doctor told me I only had two weeks to live. This was the result of cirrhosis of the liver and hepatitis C. My choices of poison were beer and champagne that I drank every night. It was normal to stop at the pub on the way home from work. I wouldn't consider myself an alcoholic but

I certainly socialised a lot. I've since found out that cirrhosis of the liver runs in my family and hepatitis C complicated my health. Looking back though, I drank socially to make myself feel more confident and fit in. I recognise now that I have a fear of walking into straight bars, and this includes socialising with straight men. In my head, I'm thinking I'll be targeted because I'm gay and I think this stems from my bullying experiences at school. Once I stopped drinking, I had to learn to embrace my fear of being ostracised as I didn't want my social life to end, so I had to dig deep and accept that my life will never be the same as it was before. I was okay with that as the alternative was death. I had a choice to make, and I chose to look after my health and really find out what makes me who I am without the beer goggles on.

What would you tell your younger self?

Take as many golden opportunities as you can when offered. I was offered hospitality positions in exotic parts of the world and I was too insecure to take them up. I, unfortunately, didn't believe I had the skills required and stayed in my comfort zone in Australia. My career history is proof that I was good enough to do the jobs overseas, but at the time my lack of confidence held me back. I regret missing out on so many adventures.

My attitude is that being gay is irrelevant as far as leading a 'normal' life goes. The only difference is that it can be a rougher ride through puberty and early manhood until you become confident in who you are.

Brad

The younger years

I grew up in the northern suburbs of Melbourne in an Australian, low socio-economic family, where luxuries were not affordable to us all the time and we lived off the welfare system. My mother has always been very supportive of me; however, I cannot say the same about my dad as he was jobless and struggled with alcoholism.

I am the youngest of three children. My older brother was like the bully; he was very misunderstood and constantly in trouble. My older sister was quite independent, so she wasn't around much when I was growing up. To be honest, I've never really had much in common with my siblings. I was always considered different.

As a nineties kid, I enjoyed watching cartoons in the morning before school, such as *Pokémon* and *Dragonball Z*, playing game boy and collecting things like Pogs or getting a Tamagotchi. Also, I remember watching a show like *Sailor Moon*, but feeling guilty about it, as it was considered by my family to be a bit too feminine. This would be the earliest memory for me about liking 'girly' stuff.

My parents were not religious at all, nor overtly homophobic, however, I do remember my father using derogatory terms when talking about gay people. Also, the same with my older brother, using references like 'that's gay' or 'what a fag'. These terms created a sense of negativity, which I believe most people can relate too.

When growing up, I had a very simplistic point of view about masculinity and femininity, such as the man was the bread winner and the woman was the homemaker.

I attended the local public schools, followed by university, where I obtained my Bachelor and Secondary Teaching DipEd. My years at high school were when I realised that I stood out as being different. I loved dressing well and wearing different types of clothing, but people considered it 'girly', alternative or punk, like the band Evanescence, so I stopped myself and dressed normal... just to conform. I was also teased for my soft tone of voice and how I stood, as my posture was perceived as 'gay', so once again I changed who I was and conformed. I concentrated on making my voice deeper, changed how I walked and stood straighter.

I liked performing in the choir and school rock bands even though that was still considered a bit artsy or gay as well. So, after a while I changed again and played more sports. I definitely preferred performing and singing to playing sports, but I reinvented myself to avoid being teased again and again.

Dating was another issue. I did date a few different girls, but I just thought they weren't my type and it didn't work out. Maybe I wasn't into it or didn't pay them enough attention. Either way, I only did it to fit in.

My peers categorised me as a typical 'gay' character as was portrayed in many movies. A singer/performer, fashionista, softly spoken man that stood 'weirdly'. There was a lot of pressure around me from my friends. Yet I still didn't understand why people thought I was gay. Looking back now, I can see I was a little different than my family and friends, and how I tried to change myself to fit in with the norms of my environment. That is how I came to understand the phrase 'we are a product of our environment'.

At my high school there were many Muslim students so it was inevitable that I would have Muslim friends. One of my closest friends was Muslim, but we never spoke about it. When I was 15 years old this religion sparked my interest, so I began to research it by reading material, going to lectures and attending the local mosque. The people at the mosque were very welcoming and kind. I felt that Islam had many positive aspects that I liked at the time. Some of these were keeping family bonds, respecting people around you, valuing things like education and practicing self-control. I was looking for these values in my own life as I had no goals or ambitions.

I made the decision to become a Muslim, which in turn gave me some order in my life and the stability I was craving. When I told my mum, her first concern was that I was being groomed to be a terrorist, but once I talked about the spiritual influence on me, she felt much better and I assured her it had nothing to do with Radicalism. After a while, I assumed Mum had told Dad about my decision to become a Muslim, but he never discussed it with me, so I thought it had been swept under the carpet as usual. He would eventually clash with me about it, questioning my beliefs and challenging me about the negative images portrayed in the media. It was difficult to defend Muslims and Islam with the generalisations and stereotypes created by society.

When I was studying at university, I met a girl named Tasniim who was also Muslim. We were both members of the Islamic Society at university and our friendship blossomed into a romance. It's traditional for women to marry within their faith and culture. I only ticked one of those boxes, which was sharing the same faith, whereas we were from different cultures. She was from Africa and I was a Caucasian Aussie. However, as time went on her family accepted me. Although, another challenge had to be faced with our union, as people would stare at us for being an interracial couple or questioning our choice of partner.

For quite some time, I was worried that my family, or mostly my father, would accidently offend my new partner. There were occasions when my dad did make some comments, while under the influence of alcohol, but Tasniim and her family were able to look past them and not take it out on me. I'm forever grateful for their understanding. Two years after meeting, we were married then had a son named Muhammad.

After all those years, I still did not consider myself to be gay or have gay tendencies, and I was quite happy and content in my marriage. The feelings of acting or looking like a typical 'gay' guy never happened again. However, in Islam, men and women are segregated a lot, so I often found myself surrounded by men. I found myself checking them out on occasions, but it never went further than that.

The realisation

At the age of 24, after finishing my course at university, I decided to travel overseas for a quick trip to visit a close friend of mine, Rasheed, who now lived in the Middle East. We were friends at university, and before he left university to move back home, I tried to encourage him to 'come out', as I was sure he was gay, but he was too scared to tell me because he thought I'd judge him. For obvious reasons, being gay and Muslim is considered haram (unlawful) and acting upon it is a sin. He spent many years living in Australia, however, he was from the Middle East, Muslim and Black. So, he faced a lot of difficulties in coming out to me, culturally and religiously.

While holidaying in the Middle East, I stayed with Rasheed at his house and he was comfortable enough to *finally* admit he was gay. We travelled around together to see the sights and hung out with his friends who identified as being discreetly homosexual. As it turned out, I got on really well with his friends and we became quite close. Again, being gay and open about it in the Middle East is a crime that can lead to jail time, deportation or death!

One day, I was having a deep and meaningful conversation with one of Rasheed's friends. We discussed all sorts of things including the topic of relationships. We talked about sexual experiences and one thing led to the other… we started kissing and I felt guilty because I was married, but not guilty for the gay behaviour. It felt very natural to me. So, I didn't feel bad for too long, but I had to stop him and left it at that as I didn't want to disrespect my wife.

Rasheed wasn't surprised about this episode and encouraged me to explore more for myself. He said his 'gaydar' was sensing

I was gay, and he felt that by being married in my early twenties, with hardly any dating experience, was the reason I never got a chance to explore my sexuality before. He suggested I go for it, but I wasn't sure myself. I liked kissing the other guy but the nagging feeling of it being bad still lingered in the back of my mind. The idea of being with a man was considered 'wrong', but that assumption is based on guilt from the prospective of others in my 'religious' circles and the stigma about what is means to be gay. I had now opened Pandora's Box giving rise to unavoidable change.

Upon my return to Australia, I ran with the mantra of 'what happens in Vegas stays in Vegas!' Married life went on as normal, except my feelings had changed in relation to how I now viewed other men. Also, the guy that I had kissed while in the Middle East, who I nicknamed Sugar, was continuing to send me flirty text messages which I enjoyed and didn't mind from time to time. However, the more interaction I had with Sugar, the less shame I had about being gay, but increased guilt because I was married. Tasniim started to question the friendships I had made in the Middle East and said I shouldn't really be friends with them. She said they seem to be gay or have gay tendencies which is against our religion. I felt she was using religious manipulation to control my friendship group and me in general.

Over the next two years our marriage slowly disintegrated as we realised we had different views on life. Even though we tried to work on our relationship, it became obvious that our marriage was not going to survive. Tasniim then suggested that I go overseas to work as a teacher where she had a contact for me to find a job, and we reached a mutual agreement to separate for a while. This gave me the opportunity to have a break from my marriage and earn good money for the family. I ended up working in the Middle East and, once again, catching up with Rasheed.

He knew my marriage was on the rocks and suggested that I start exploring dating sites like Grindr or Hornet. This is a path that I wanted to go down to see if I was really gay, as I still wasn't 100 per cent convinced. I ended up meeting an Arab man named Ahmed. He was sweet, a joker and educated. He made me feel comfortable and we enjoyed each other's company. He was the first man I ever liked enough to consider having a relationship with. Unfortunately, living overseas as an expat is short lived. I was 27 years old and not enjoying the job I had in the Middle East. Ahmed and I both agreed to move on, so I returned home to Australia. I tried saving my marriage, but it was too toxic and not salvageable. The end result was divorce. I was now in a position where I found myself free and alone to explore who I am without any restrictions connected to marriage or religion.

I decided to relocate back to the Middle East and live closer to Rasheed. He was super supportive which helped me to feel comfortable with my return to living overseas. As soon as I landed in my new apartment, I perused the dating apps to check in and see who was around me. Obviously, being new to the area, many guys were messaging me (it was a good ego boost). The first person who messaged me was a man named Yazan. We hit it off immediately and decided to meet up at my apartment the next day. He showed up at my place in a traditional Arabian outfit, wearing sunglasses and an Arabian head piece. I started to laugh out loud and said to him, 'Does that work for all the whites you meet?' He laughed nervously, and I proceeded to show him all my Arabian outfits that I wore to attend mosque for Friday prayers. He was visibly shocked and couldn't understand how a white Australian had integrated himself into Arabic culture.

We sat down, and I explained everything about myself and my life before coming to the Middle East.

From that day forward, Yazan and myself have been together and have never been apart until many years later. We decided to become partners in 2018 and started to work on an Australian marriage visa. At the end of 2019, I moved back to Australia due to COVID-19, and I'm sad to say that we have been separated since. It's now March 2021 without any hint of seeing each other for a while yet.

Coming out

None of my friends had any concerns about me being gay, but I still hadn't told my family. I thought I'd start with my mum. When I returned from the Middle East for a holiday in 2017, it was around the time of the Marriage Equality referendum, and I was pleasantly surprised at how accepting and supportive the general population were of the LGBTIQ community. Even when I went to the AFL, there were rainbow flags everywhere, social media was supportive, as were the media at large.

At the same time, I had a close friend from Pakistan called Zohaib, who was encouraging me to tell my mum. He was not able to tell his own family, and he wished he was able to have the opportunity that I had. He said, 'They are white and Australian, are you stupid?!' For some reason, I had the Muslim mentality of not being accepted for being gay from my family. His straight forwardness gave me a wakeup call! He was right! My mum is Aussie and she would be more accepting compared to other people. Zohaib really wanted me to be freer than he will ever be with expressing his sexuality to family. I will always have gratitude for his words and friendship.

Zohaib had given me the courage to make the decision to tell my mum. I arranged a dinner with her at a restaurant so we could talk candidly. To get the conversation started, I brought up the topic of the Referendum to use as a segue. Using humour as a defence mechanism, I proceeded to make a joke about what she would say if I brought a guy home. This is how I deal with awkward moments. Mum laughed and said, 'That would be funny.' I then launched into telling her on a more serious note, that actually I would like to bring someone home. She said, 'Wait, what?', with a surprised look on her face. I then said, 'Because I have found someone who makes me really happy and he lives overseas.' She hesitated and said, 'He?' I now had a tear running down my face. I explained to her that I was in love with a man named Yazan. He is from the Middle East and he's the reason I have been staying there for so long. Mum said that she's happy for me as she knows how unhappy I was in my marriage and only wants to see me happy. She did suggest I don't tell Dad because he has such a big mouth. She then went on and changed the subject, which made me feel a little let down because it was so... anticlimactic, as there was such a build up to telling her (I was expecting a bit more drama). As it turned out, I didn't have to worry as Mum has been supportive of me ever since. I'm grateful the outcome has been a positive one, as there are many people, especially Muslims, who don't get this support in life.

About three years later, in 2019, I had returned to Australia and was no longer living in the Middle East. I was having a conversation with my dad, who was now separated from my mum and living in his own apartment block. He started talking to me about a person living in his apartment block, and referred to him as a 'faggot', and this triggered me. So, in anger, I said, 'How would you feel if you use that language, knowing that people would not want to approach you? It makes it hard to chat with a bigot! Well, I'm gay, so what do you think about that?' Dad began to backpedal really fast, even his voice changed as he told me he's accepting of homosexuals and had friends that were gay. He said he didn't mean to be homophobic and he does accept me. There was not much conversation after that and we talked about other things. I found it hard to believe him. Telling my dad was probably my biggest moment of coming out, as I didn't know how he would respond. I was proud that I was able to express myself without thinking about the consequences. As he was known for being a big gossip; he probably would've done me a favour as I no longer had to tell the rest of the family – he'd sort that out real quick!

Moving forward, I feel like I haven't fully 'come out' as yet because I'm more of a private person. I believe people don't necessarily need to know about such feelings or identities, unless it was brought up in conversation. I have accepted who I am and my sexuality, however, I've learnt to read the room and my audience, so I only reveal this side of me when it's appropriate or when I'm in the mood. Also, because of the limitations of being a gay Muslim, I'm guarded when in the presence of my Muslim community for fear of being judged and ostracised. This is not just about protecting myself; it extends to other people in my friendship groups and especially my son.

Life after coming out

After coming out, there was a sense of relief and acceptance as now I don't have to be so guarded around my family. My parents divorced after I was divorced. I believe it gave my mum the courage to do it after seeing me go through the process and thriving. Mum and I have become closer and have been concentrating on our health and fitness since I came out. She has gone on to become a teacher's assistant and is also working for the NDIS. I have been living with Mum since returning from the Middle East in 2019, and we have become great supports for each other.

Currently, I am communicating with Yazan. He is still living in the Middle East due to COVID-19, so I haven't seen him since returning to Australia. We had been together since 2015, but due to him having a Yemeni passport, he's been unable to get a visa, even as a tourist. This is purely based on him being rejected by the Australian government, as they view him as a potential asylum seeker. This is not the case, but very hard to prove otherwise. I'm finding it quite difficult to support him as we're running out of avenues to pursue, so our lives together are very up in the air at the moment.

To apply for an Australian Partnership Visa, there is much evidence that needs to be provided to prove that we're a committed couple with years of history together. We lived together for three years or more before I returned to Australia, but because we are not married (this applies to straight and gay people), a rented apartment in the Middle East can only be registered in the name of an individual or in joint names as a married couple. This makes it extremely difficult to prove that we are in a committed relationship.

Also, because we are Muslim and living in a country where being gay is a crime, we were never able to make our relationship public. This meant no photos relating to our relationship such as going out for dinner to celebrate an anniversary, changing my relationship status to 'in a relationship' on Facebook, no holiday or other couple photos of us on Instagram. I eventually managed to create a private account for ourselves to post images that included close friends and other gay people within our circle. Sometimes, this is risky to do, but we want to show that we are in love and are able to express that like everyone else. In reality, there is no paper or electronic evidence that we are a couple. Our life together in the Middle East can only exist in our memories – nothing tangible or as solid as people living in countries that accept gay rights. We had to lead a very discreet life where all evidence of our relationship had to be hidden. Like most people who identify as gay in the Middle East, these are the challenges faced.

All evidence has to be secret. This makes it very difficult to prove that we are in a committed relationship. We've hired an immigration lawyer to work on our behalf, but their priority due to COVID-19, are couples that are already landside, meaning onshore, or already living in Australia. Currently, Partner Visas offshore are not a priority. It's extremely frustrating but Yazan and I are determined to be together. It's been a long and hard journey for us, and at times, we've had discussions around moving on to find other partners, but we're not sure. We're currently in an open relationship, but I struggle with being alone and so far away from him. I have met other people for friendship and/or fun, and it sometimes crosses my mind that perhaps I could move on from Yazan, but I feel it wouldn't be fair. I probably need to move on fully and not lead others on.

Influences in search of happiness

On my quest in the pursuit of happiness, especially in the gay community, I had to find people who I could be myself around, relax with and talk about any subject whether it was personal or not, and with no judgement. I had that support network when living in the Middle East with people like Rasheed, Zohaib and Yazan, but once I returned to Australia leaving everyone behind, I've had to begin all over again to build a family of friends that provide support and comradery in Australia, otherwise, I would feel very much alone. Even though my immediate family accepts me, they don't understand or are capable of discussing the deeper issues that I've had to deal with. I've travelled down life paths that are so far removed from their lives. The groups of people I associate with are the gay community and Muslim community to which they have very little understanding or experience of each other. This is why it's been so important for me to find like-minded people to enhance my joy and happiness in life.

Biggest challenges in life

I find there is pressure from the gay community to be openly gay and shout it from the rooftops, but as I'm quite a private person, I do not believe that is necessary. Being Muslim and openly 'out' is not common. There are two other areas that I'm challenged in: one is in the Muslim community and the other is with those who are non-Muslim.

I'm challenged by the Muslim community to not 'out' myself for fear of rejection, and then when non-Muslims know I'm gay, there is pressure to constantly explain my position as a gay Muslim. I also feel the need to defend the Muslim community to the gay community in regard to their beliefs, as they are entitled to their faith, even though I don't fit the mould.

One of my biggest fears is that my son will be ostracised by the Muslim community if they find out his father is gay. Mind you, my son knows I'm gay and I've warned him not to talk about my sexuality, as he could also be bullied for it. It makes me sad that he has to keep this secret, but my hope for him is that he will grow up in the next generation as a voice of understanding and tolerance for all.

Unfortunately, I still feel like I'm living a double life. The gay community is encouraging me to be more open, yet, within the Muslim community I'm still hiding – it's a 'catch-22' situation. This is the struggle a lot of gay Muslims have to face. This is why the family of friends I build around me are so important as a practical solution, so I don't go mad with constantly having to be discreet or not having people to relate too.

Another layer to my challenges, is the subject of homosexuality as it's constantly under scrutiny in the Muslim community when there are much more pressing problems in the world. In argument, I've brought up examples of other more problematic issues in the Muslim world that is considered a sin, such as adultery, drugs, stealing, lying and alcohol. One of the worst sins is Riba (interest, exploitation gains in trade or dealings, especially linked to home loans in the Islamic community) which are also considered a sin in the Qur'an. It seems these issues are treated more lightly, even though they are prevalent in the Muslim community whereas being gay is viewed as much more serious. Overall, their reasoning is that there is too much homosexuality in the world and it will take over. Funnily enough, this is the same argument a racist would say about Muslims coming over to steal their jobs by migrating to Australia. So, what to do?

What would you tell your younger self?

Don't change a thing about yourself. But as a heads up, don't be so hard on yourself and have some patience (in Arabic – sabr) as things in life don't always happen when you want them to. You will eventually find the place where you belong, even though you could be challenged multiple times for being different. It will all work out in the end, just have some faith.

Scott

The younger years

For the past 13 years I've been living in Australia but I grew up in the UK in a city called Norwich. Norwich was a manufacturing town for shoes and was located in a fairly isolated part of England.

I was from a working-class family. My parents were not well educated and even though they worked really hard, they still struggled financially and there was little money for any luxuries. Dad worked through the day for an electricity company, while Mum stayed home to look after myself and my brother, Andrew. She then went to work at night in a shoe factory on a processing line while our dad cared for us.

As a child, I always enjoyed learning, so early on, school was a highlight for me as I found it easy to achieve high grades. Unfortunately, I was bullied frequently when I attended high school. It was emotional bullying mainly, and to add insult to injury, it was my friends that I had in junior school who then became my tormenters in high school, led by their new friends. My grades suffered as a result, as did my emotional health. My parents did the best they could with the knowledge and experience they had in regard to the bullying. Mum would write me absentee notes for school when I was feeling overwhelmed by the bullying. I'm sure she felt absolutely helpless as to how to deal with this situation, whereas my dad was brought up in an era where you were told to fight back, so that was the only solution he could give me. He was from the school of hard knocks and couldn't relate to my sensitive nature. I, however, was not a fighter, so I was left feeling alone with no one to talk to. I felt unsupported by him, but I see now that he didn't have the emotional intelligence to deal with my feelings as he was old school.

I didn't know anyone who was gay. My father was openly homophobic. He would refer to homosexuals as 'poofs' and he was clearly not comfortable with the idea of gay people. Nothing was ever said directly to me when I was young, however, I sensed that they believed it was not acceptable or normal. These views were not related to religion; to them it was just abnormal. I have vivid memories of the Grim Reaper advertisements on TV in the eighties during the AIDS epidemic, and my family vocalised that the gays deserved to get AIDS because of who they were and their lifestyle. They were not sympathetic at all!

The realisation

I was about six years old when I went to a holiday camp with my family, and I was quite taken with the male archery instructor. It wasn't sexual, but there was a feeling I couldn't quite understand at such a young age, although I instinctively knew it was an attraction.

The life model that I grew up with was the traditional family of marrying a girl, having children and living in our own home. I didn't believe there were any other options. Despite having an attraction towards men from the age of 17 years, I did have girlfriends. My first love was Eliza. We were together from the age of 17 to 22 – we got engaged and lived together. When I was 22, I purchased my first computer. I was curious about how I was feeling so I started to ask questions in gay forums and websites. At no time did I ever cheat on Eliza when we were together. After a time, I came to the conclusion that I couldn't continue the lie anymore, and that it wasn't only my life I was affecting. She wanted to have children and the thought of what is considered the traditional life, was now no longer an option for me.

It all came to a head one night when I ended up in tears as I couldn't hold it in for one more second. Eliza asked me what was wrong, and I went on to tell her I don't feel the same way about her as she did for me, and she deserved better. I didn't have the courage to tell her I was gay. I felt so guilty that I gave her everything that we owned together including an extra lump sum of money. Eliza did move on to get married and have two children, but I believe she is now divorced.

My first gay sexual encounter was with a man and his boyfriend I met through a chat room. I travelled 65 km to meet them. Although I was incredibly nervous, it was a positive experience and it affirmed for me that my sexual preference was men, not women. It was not long after this, that I then decided to move to Jersey in the Channel Islands after a suggestion from a friend who lived there. As it turned out, Jersey was similar to Norwich: small, insular and most gays were still in the closet which made it more difficult to come out than if I resided in London. But it was here that I really started to accept myself and get comfortable with being gay.

Coming out

I made the best friends of my life after I left Norwich. I didn't have to hide anymore, the bullying was behind me and I was away from the small mindedness, although, I was still fearful of telling my parents that I was gay due to their homophobic mentality. I was tired of leading a double life as I had been living with my boyfriend, Jay, for two years at this point, and not able to talk about the relationship with my family. By this time, I was 28 years old and ready to come out. I decided to tell Mum first, but not until I plied her with a few drinks. I still found it extremely hard to actually say that I was gay. Just saying the word 'gay' would get stuck in my throat. I started the conversation with, 'You know Jay isn't my flatmate, Mum?' to which she replied, 'Scott, are you gay?', and I replied with a 'yes'. She then went on to say that they thought I was, but because I had been engaged to Eliza, they were thrown off the scent. Mum told Dad after I left that night. Initially, he told me it would take some time to get used to the idea, but he very quickly became cool with it all, and openly expressed interest in meeting my partner.

Quite soon after coming out, Mum and Dad visited me in London so they could meet Jay. It was nerve wracking for me as it's one thing to announce you're gay, but it's another to introduce your parents to your partner. As it turned out, I had nothing to worry about as they fell in love with Jay, and my mum was ecstatic that she didn't have to worry about the possible tension that can come from having a daughter-in-law. My parents were heart broken when I broke up with Jay after 12 years, and to this day, Jay and my mum are still in contact.

My dad's attitude toward the gay community completely changed. If he hears someone talking in derogatory terms about gays, he is very quick to defend them now, and he's extremely proud of me. For someone who's not really in touch with his feelings and is a man of few words, it's nice to know he's got my back.

Life after coming out

For me it was utter relief as I no longer had to live two separate lives. The feelings of being deceitful were eradicated as I didn't have to be concerned anymore about getting tripped up or caught out in a lie. Because I was already living as a gay man with my partner in London away from family before I came out, life didn't actually change much except that now when my parents visited me more in London, the stress of lying was gone. At a level, I became closer to my parents and I was able to give them an education into my gay world.

In 2009, Jay was offered a job in Sydney and we decided it would be a great adventure to make the move together. Unfortunately, our relationship did not last, and in 2015 we broke up. I now call Australia home – I am an Australian Citizen and I own my own business here. Our relationship was the instigator for me living a lifestyle I could only have dreamt of.

Influences in search of happiness

When I was 23 and living in Jersey, I was in a relationship with a much older guy, Chris, who was 40 years old. He was kind of my sugar daddy for a while, but I'll forever be grateful for what I learnt from him, as he protected me and was generous and kind. We were together for about six months then became very good friends after that, until he passed away five years later from suicide. I have such fond memories of our time together. He flew us to London where I went to my first gay nightclub called, Heaven, and it was like heaven for me. It was so over the top with hot guys everywhere and I felt completely at home compared to Jersey or Norwich, where there was no gay scene. Chris helped me navigate the ins and outs of gay life as I was rather naïve to the ways of the world. I realise now, he was a bit of a father figure to me as I felt I didn't have a close relationship with my own father at the time. He opened my eyes to a world I hadn't known existed before, which gave me the confidence to go to London to study. This was his gift to me.

I'm extremely fortunate to be surrounded by friends who have supported me through all my ups and downs in life. Jay taught me about true love, companionship and depth of connection that I haven't felt since we broke up six years ago. Ryan, who is also from the UK and lives in Australia, is like a brother to me who is also gay, so it's an easy friendship where no topic is off the table. Our outlook on life is similar as is our background, and I think we're cut from the same cloth. This is a friendship that I truly cherish. I believe I've finally found my tribe.

Biggest challenges in life

I think my biggest challenge is accepting that I'm allowed to be me. I've never felt overly comfortable with the gay culture. I dress fairly conservatively, I'm not interested in party drugs, open relationships or living a hedonistic lifestyle, even my career as a physiotherapist is mainstream. I would consider myself to be a straight-acting gay man. Trying to fit in with this culture has created much anxiety and depression within myself and the wider gay community, due to the pressure of acting and behaving in a certain way. I believe everyone should live their life how they want to live it, but the stereotypical gay life as portrayed in the media is not my thing.

The vote for marriage equality in Australia affected me much more than I thought it would. This is a decision that should have been made by politicians and not gone to a referendum. It's bad enough being made to feel different than heterosexual people, then to highlight the differences, by asking the population of Australia to vote on whether same sex marriage should be legal or not. Whilst it opened up a dialogue, it also drew out the haters and religious fanatics who spewed their righteous beliefs in a very public forum. Luckily, the outcome was positive, but I shudder to think if this had gone the other way, how much more damage would have been done to the LGBTIQ community!

Another challenge I seem to face is the feeling that I'm constantly having to come out. Every time someone asks me if I'm married or why don't I have a girlfriend, I feel pressured to say why, but I don't think it's any of their business. This makes me feel awkward, and sometimes I just lie and say I haven't met the right one yet. For me it's easier that way, however, I'd rather not be put in a position to have to explain myself over and over. If I were straight, I'd never have to feel awkward if someone asked me that question as there would be no fear of judgement. As a gay man, I am often wary of people's judgements, and I don't want to set myself up to be judged.

What would you tell your younger self?

In my mind, I assumed that my parents had expectations of how I should live, and I conformed to their way of thinking. In doing this, I didn't trust my own feelings; consequently, I lived a lie for many years. If only I had realised my family would have loved me regardless, I could have saved myself much angst.

If I had followed my intuition and been brave enough to do what I wanted to do with my life, I wouldn't have suffered so much emotional turmoil. As I get older, I'm becoming more comfortable in my own skin and it's a nice place to be.

Do not wait until you're at breaking point before putting your needs and wants first because you are the most important person in your life – with no exceptions!

Troy

The younger years

I was the youngest of three children with an older brother and sister, and we grew up in Toowoomba with Mum and Dad. From a very young age, my dad physically abused me as he was an alcoholic. This abuse didn't stop until I was 16 years old, as I became stronger and was able to stand up to him. He never hit my mum, but he constantly abused us kids, both emotionally and physically. To the outside world he was a cool guy; all the extended family and friends loved him as he would drink and was fun to be around. Behind the scenes though, he was an evil person who couldn't hold his liquor. He would come home drunk from the pub and throw the meal that Mum had made him against the wall. That is only one example of his appalling behaviour. I was scared of my dad, as he knew I was different from other kids and we had very little in common. My father used to say to people when I was younger, 'I have a son, a daughter and Troy.' Meaning that he didn't acknowledge me as his son which really hurt when growing up. He had a sense that I was gay, long before I did, which didn't help our relationship. Consequently, I don't have many fond memories of my childhood.

It was Mum who taught me what love was, but even that came crashing down. When I was 11 years old, I caught Mum having an affair with Dad's best friend. She forced me to keep the secret until the affair was finally out in the open when I was 16. Being forced to keep this secret destroyed the trust I had in my mum. The lesson I took away from those turbulent times was that those who love you are the ones that hurt you. This thinking does not set you up to live a happy life!

My saving grace was my interest in the art and drama subjects at school. As I loved performing in musicals at the local theatre, at the age of 17 I auditioned for a drama college in Brisbane, to which I was accepted. Even though I was now exposed to the gay lifestyle, unlike in Toowoomba back in the eighties, it still didn't click in me the fact that I had gay tendencies. Even when I was growing up my brother and random people would call me a 'poofter'. I hated being labelled; I still do, as I'm just me.

When I was 18, I met my future wife Sarah and we were married four years later. She was a strong woman who stood up for and supported me. She was able to look after me like I hadn't been looked after before, and she taught me strength while I taught her to mind her tongue. It could be a bit toxic at times. We had what I would consider a normal sexual relationship with no gay thoughts on my behalf. Looking back, I realise now I had more female friends than male friends. After I was married, I didn't talk to my dad for two-and-a-half years which helped me grow in confidence without his negative input. I was determined to be successful in my career and life to prove to my family I was successful and worthy.

The realisation

Sarah and I tried to have a baby for five years, and finally, at the age of 29, we had a son. I was now committed to a family and house mortgage. It made me think, what the hell am I doing, do I really want this? I felt trapped! It was not long after this realisation when I was on the train going to work, I happened to meet a guy called Gary. We started chatting and seemed to hit it off immediately with lots in common. He was also married with children and our families became good friends, even to the point where we holidayed together. Unbeknownst to anyone else, Gary and I had an affair for 13 years, until I began looking around at other men.

Incredulously, I still didn't consider myself gay!

I realised that it was intimacy that I missed with both Sarah and Gary. Looking back, I was in absolute denial. With Gary it was a relationship without all the usual commitments. After 21 years of marriage, I broke up with Sarah, and also with Gary. The reason I gave to Sarah about breaking up was not that I was gay, but that I was not in love with her anymore. For me that was the truth at the time. I then decided to move to the Sunshine Coast for a fresh start. This was a massive change for me. I finally felt free and able to do whatever I want by exploring the world around me. I jumped feet first into online chat rooms. This is where I met Thomas, who I proceeded to see for about two months, but I still felt like I was missing out on the intimacy. This was the turning point for me, when I finally acknowledged to myself that I was gay and there was no denying it. I enjoyed the feel, touch and company of being with a man. I wanted just one, not heaps of men as I needed security and love.

Coming out

My coming out was a big 'oops' moment! I had sent messages to Thomas, not knowing that the messages were diverting to Sarah's iPad. This is how she found out and for some reason, once she realised I was gay, she wanted me back. I realised Thomas wasn't right for me and I questioned did I want a gay relationship. Upon reflection he was the wrong person for me. Unexplainably, I returned to Toowoomba and the marriage for two-and-a-half years where I easily slipped right back in to the marriage, as if I had never left.

Life after coming out

Only one friend of ours in Toowoomba knew of my past, so it was quite easy to return to my marriage even though I was officially 'out'. Occasionally, Sarah would throw it back in my face and as time went on, our relationship turned into a friendship as we were only living together with no intimacy at all. In that time after I returned, I did not cheat on Sarah. She actually said I could do what I needed to do, but she didn't want to know about it. We played our roles and pretended that everything was fine, when it so was not.

In 2017, after my father passed away, I learned how miserable my parents were as my mother finally divulged the news that they should have broken up long ago. This was the catalyst that made me realise how unhappy I was with my life. I returned to living a gay lifestyle even though I was still living with Sarah. The mask could now come off once and for all. I sat down and told her that I was now having sex with guys and this was how I wanted to live my life moving forward. I reinforced that I wanted to be with someone who I could have a committed relationship with.

Eventually we agreed that we were both unhappy. I needed intimacy and fun in my life and I couldn't do that with a woman. I felt I had to give it one more try with Sarah, but it only lasted six weeks. I had lots of fun and sex with Sarah, but how was this going to work moving forward? The short answer was: it wasn't going to work. It cemented the fact that I couldn't have a full relationship if I stayed with her. She was really upset, but came to accept that it wasn't going to work and I asked for a divorce. I lived on my own for three months after the separation. When I told my son that I was gay, he was 19 years old at the time. He understood that I wanted intimacy but didn't quite understand why I was with a man. To a certain degree he has accepted that I'm gay – thank goodness.

I was now 49 years old and ready to start my new life on my terms. It was around this time that I met a guy called Kurt. We clicked from the get-go which made me think that I really wanted a relationship with him, as did he. We dated for a while, then he moved in with me as Kurt had broken up with his previous partner who he was sharing an apartment with. It was refreshing to be able to take my mask off and not lie anymore. Being honest with myself has liberated me. I now realise, that for me, life is all about being wanted and loved. In hindsight, I probably should have had a bit more time on my own to work on who I am and what I'm about. I quickly jumped into a relationship only three months after fully coming out and I lost a little bit of who I am. However, I'm happy in my relationship with Kurt.

Influences in search of happiness

I attended a funeral with Kurt for one of his family members, and this was the first time I met his whole family. I have to admit I was quite nervous at the start, but to my surprise, I couldn't believe how well they accepted me. I felt like it was the first time I could be myself with a gay partner in public, because I could be my normal self around them. It was very comforting as I've always craved that. I will be forever thankful to his family for welcoming and accepting me so graciously into their lives. We have been the voice of reason for each other's families and have brought them all together.

It was at this time that I came out to my friends and family. The first person I told was a work colleague who was fully supportive. This reaction gave me the courage to tell my mum. I decided to visit her so I could tell her in person. When I rang Mum to tell her I was coming down to visit, she asked me, 'Is Kurt your true friend?', to which I replied, 'What do you mean?' She said, 'Is he your partner?', and I replied, 'Yes.' Mum went on to say, 'I thought so.' And in the background, I could hear my sister yell out, 'I told you he was!' Here I was thinking I'd pulled the wool over their eyes. Over a period of a few months, I slowly came out to people I knew and no one judged me as I had feared – not one person put me down. They were all very supportive. The weight off my shoulders was massive because it was only a big deal to me and no one else. I shouldn't have been so worried or scared, their love didn't change for me as no one treated me differently. I am me and was finally accepted as me.

Biggest challenges in life

Once I took the masks off, which was very liberating, I felt much more vulnerable and more easily hurt than before. Nothing left to hide behind now. Not that I would go back, I just need to learn how to deal with these new feelings and increase my resilience.

Another challenge I have is allowing myself to be happy now that I'm out, as I wasn't sure how to do that before. I'm still trying to sort out if it's relationship issues or working out who I am as a gay man. I've had to grow emotionally and find myself for me to become stronger as a person, in order for me to know who I am and what I want in life. I've struggled with this a bit as I'm also working out who I am while in a new relationship, which is difficult for anyone to do, let alone a man who's recently come out.

Add to this, I recognise that I'm terrified to be on my own which has been a struggle for me all my life. This explains why I've stayed in bad relationships far too long – 'better the devil you know' attitude. Feeling wanted all the time is a challenge for me and wanting things to be perfect in life. Maybe there's a touch of OCD in there! I felt like my life had flatlined after coming out as there is such a build up to coming out, and then it's, 'Oh, is that it?' Back to reality. I'm happy though because I can now see me.

COVID times have put pressure on my relationship with Kurt, as I have much more time to think about things and haven't been distracted with going out and having fun. I've struggled with the restrictions as I can't go out and dance and experience parts of the gay culture. Instead, it feels like we have turned into old married men mode, but I am embracing that now. Life will return to normal soon so we can experience life together.

Another challenge I've had is friends telling me that I shouldn't have jumped so quickly into a long-term relationship after coming out. I'm not interested in having lots of flings, so what's the issue if I've found someone that I click with who makes me happy? I'm now a bit wary of telling friends if I've had words with Kurt, as they're quick to tell me I shouldn't be in another relationship so soon. I believe each to their own as I'm the only one who knows what's right for me, even if I do have to find out the hard way.

What would you tell your younger self?

Do not settle if it doesn't feel right!

Give yourself time to find out who you really are, what you want and why, rather than rushing in and filling a gap in your life with meaningless stuff or experiences.

Being gay doesn't mean that you have to be alone with no family. You can accept a partner's family or friends' families, as people in general are much more accepting these days.

In the past, I thought that if I came out, I would have to move to another city, but times have changed and I've been pleasantly surprised as the world didn't blow up in my face.

You don't have to wear a label; be you. I am me. Love me or hate me, I am who I am and I'm proud! I deserve happiness, fulfilment and love.

Anne Considine – my story

I'll start from when Chris was eight years old. My husband, Paul, was so excited that he had two sons to play footy with, starting with Vickick (as it was called in the mid-nineties, it's now Auskick). When they returned home from the first session, Paul said, 'Anne, I don't think Chris is that interested in football. When the boys were running around after the ball, Chris was down the other end of the oval with another boy digging a hole in the ground!' He went on to say, 'That's okay, as long as he's not gay!' Not a word of a lie. He was joking at the time, but I did hear him make that remark occasionally over the next five years or so, and that is when a joke stops being a joke. Keep in mind that Paul came from a strict Catholic family, he played football at the highest level with Hawthorn and he worked in the family transport company. All very blokey and religious. He was definitely homophobic, but would never say anything to hurt anyone deliberately. So, after hearing this remark a few times, I pulled him up one day and said, 'Paul, if any of our children are gay, don't make me choose between you and them, as I will always choose them over you, just letting you know.' He didn't say anything to that and life went on as normal.

Fast forward about seven years, Chris was now 19 and making the most of being an adult and enjoying socialising – way too much for our liking! He had the odd girlfriend when he was younger but nothing serious, which is why we didn't really pick up that he was gay. We didn't get to have the conversation that starts with, 'Mum and Dad I have something to tell you.' Chris enlisted his younger sister, Laura, to set us up by planting a thought in our head so that we would initiate the question, 'Are you gay?' He told Laura that if we asked him, he wouldn't lie. It was a Friday afternoon when I was driving Laura somewhere, she was 15 at the time, and she asked me if I thought Chris was gay. I thought this an odd question out of the blue and said something along the lines of, 'I don't think so but if he is it's okay and why do you ask?' Laura just shrugged it off with a reply of, 'No real reason,' and we left it at that. I forgot about it until a few days later on the Sunday when I told Paul. We had a bit of a discussion about it but until there was anything concrete to discuss, we moved onto other things.

Now, Chris was one for pushing boundaries. He would go out on Friday night and not return until sometime on Sunday which drove us absolutely mad, as all we needed was a text message to say he was okay. The conversation with Laura on the Friday was one of those weekends when Chris was who knows where. On that Sunday night, about an hour before friends were coming over to watch a big footy match with us between Hawthorn and Collingwood, Chris rolls in the door. We'd had enough, and so we sat him down for the chat about matters including showing respect to us. Once the lecture was over, we told him to have a shower and get ready for our guests' arrival. As he walked out of the room, Paul says to me, do you think he is gay? I said I'd go and ask him. I found Chris, as usual, with his head stuck in the pantry ferreting for food. I told him about Laura's question to me and his response was to laugh. I actually turned him around to look at me and I asked the question, 'Are you gay?', to which he replied, 'Yes.' I took a deep breath then said, 'Are you sure?!' It's quite funny looking back now, as it was a knee jerk reaction. Paul and I had a quick chat with Chris before everyone arrived, but I couldn't even tell you what it was about – our heads were spinning! That evening was bit of a blur as we were shell shocked to say the least as we tried to get our heads around this information that had just been divulged. I went into protection mode as a mum for Chris, while Paul dealt with the internal struggle of having a gay son that went against all that he had been taught as a Catholic. Fortunately, he put his son first and continued to love him and accept him as much as he did before, while trying his hardest not to judge him. It took a while, but he got there in the end and I didn't have to choose between my husband and children. I was more concerned with the lifestyle that Chris was leading. He went down the typical path of partying, drugs and alcohol and getting lost in the pleasure-seeking side of gay life. I know that not all gay men venture down this path, but it's so common. Thank goodness he is now well and truly out the other side, having partied hard and survived.

It was about six years later that Anthony, our second son, came out. Believe it or not, it was not any easier to come to terms with. At the time, Paul probably wondered why he was dealt this hand in life and I, once again, went into protective mode. But the difference this time for me, was the realisation that I probably won't be surrounded by lots of grandchildren as I imagined myself to be, having had three children of my own. My future dreams shifted somewhat, and I had to keep reminding myself that this wasn't about me, it was about the boys being happy and well adjusted. Much to Laura's horror, I laughingly told her she now has to have six children to make up for the boys in case they don't adopt! But seriously, at the end of the day, what makes me happy is having happy and well-adjusted children no matter how they decide to live their lives or who they love. Paul has since said that the best thing that ever happened to him was having two gay sons. It has taught him what is important in life and how to love unconditionally. We are grateful for the beautiful family we have, and we think that it's actually an improved version of what we thought it may have been in the past.

As a little side note, there are moments in life that warm your heart and everything is right with the world. Here are a couple to do with my boys. I was watching the movie P.S. I Love You one day with Chris and as we were watching, both of us agreed on how gorgeous Gerard Butler is. We then went on to have a chat about what physical features Chris likes in a man. He immediately said, 'muscles', to which I replied, 'Me too!', as we both laughed out loud. Another day I walked into the house and I could see Chris and Laura outside sunbaking by the pool with their heads close together in deep conversation. I wandered out and said, 'What are you two up to?' They both looked up and said, 'We're talking about our boyfriend problems.' I loved it! And Anthony has kept us entertained with funny stories of various dates he's been on. It doesn't get much better than that; my children talking about normal things in life such as careers, relationships, socialising and enjoying each other's company. But what really excites me is that there are no secrets and the kids can just be themselves.

Dianne –
Lindsay's mother

Lindsay has already told his story in this book, and he asked me if I would like to tell my experience of him coming out. I feel privileged that he asked me to contribute my story.

I didn't pick that Lindsay was gay. To me, he was as 'normal' as any other kid. We live in the small country town of Warracknabeal, and it was expected that he would play football. He definitely gave it a go to please his father, but he didn't like playing the game, so I suggested he play hockey. This is when the slurs of being gay started, as hockey was considered a gay sport for boys. To his credit, he continued to play hockey as he enjoyed it much more than football.

Lindsay was a people pleaser, and I used to say to him, the people you usually try to please are not the ones that you should be pleasing. They tend to be the ones that you're trying to impress or fit in with. He has such a kind heart, but it may also be his undoing as he could be taken advantage of.

Lindsay attended a private school for approximately 18 months, and one day I was driving him back to school after the holidays, and he was in tears all the way. I asked him what was wrong. He said he didn't want to go back, but did not say why. Consequently, he finished Year 12 back at home, as I couldn't stand to see him so unhappy.

Once he finished his secondary education, Lindsay worked in Warracknabeal at the Yarriambiack Shire Council, but was quite bored in this job as he needs to be challenged, but he wasn't. He decided to move to Melbourne for work in the hospitality industry, which he loved and was very capable. I used to travel down to Melbourne on a fairly regular basis with a girlfriend to shop, and this is when I would catch up with Lindsay. One day he rang me to see when I was visiting next. I happened to be planning a trip on my own this time, to which he seemed to be pleased, even though he is very fond of my girlfriend that I usually travel with. When we caught up for a drink, he seemed quite nervous. He said he had something to tell me; immediately my heart began to beat a bit faster. He then went on to tell me he was gay. And here am I thinking that he was going to tell me something terrible. I almost gave a sigh of relief, and had no problem accepting my son. I just wanted him to be happy. Lindsay was worried that I would be upset that he wouldn't be able to give me grandchildren, but I told him that I didn't have children to have grandchildren, so that was not an issue for me. He was not keen to tell his father, so I suggested I take on that role as I knew his father, Mick, wouldn't take it well. It seemed like a very long drive home to Warracknabeal after Lindsay's news, as I still had to digest what he had told me.

Not long after I arrived back in Warracknabeal, I arranged for Mick to call in on his way home from work, as we were separated by then. After a bit of chit chat, I told him that Lindsay was gay. His reaction was shock and annoyance. He tried to blame everyone else for 'making' Lindsay gay. He carried on by trying to blame a teacher at school who was gay and society in general with their liberal views. He then went on to say, 'There was no one gay when I went to school,' to which I replied, 'I'm sure there was, they just hadn't come out.' I also told him that Lindsay is the same person as he was last week, and he hasn't changed just because he's told us he's gay. It didn't matter what I said, there was no appeasing him, so I sent him on his way as nothing positive was coming out of his mouth. I did ring Mick a few times to make sure he was okay. He was still reeling from the news and couldn't quite come to terms with it. Their relationship wasn't close anyway, and this certainly didn't bring them any closer together – quite the opposite! Lindsay will never be able to live up to his unrealistic expectations.

I didn't realise there was worse news to come! On another trip to Melbourne and catching up with Lindsay, he went on to tell me he had a drug habit, but was functioning well and to not worry, and also not to ring him every day to see how he was. So, I had another very long trip home to Warracknabeal where I cried all the way. After much thought, I rang him the next day and told him he couldn't dump that news on me and tell me not to talk to him about it. He must have mulled it over, and he made the decision to return home to get clean. We did lots of walking and talking (sometimes in silence) and eating healthily to help him get back on track. He succeeded for a while, but the demons returned and the temptation became too much, resulting in him using again. Not long after his return to drugs, he took off from home to Melbourne without telling anyone. This was the time I thought I had lost my son forever! All sorts of horrible scenarios were going through my mind – I was absolutely distraught. A few days later, he finally got in touch with me and decided to come back home.

When he felt strong enough to return to Melbourne (Warracknabeal was too small for him), he did succeed in staying clean for a period of time, but he was easily led, and once again ended up slipping back into old habits. He evidently got into trouble with the Police over drugs, as talked about in his story, but he didn't tell me until six months after the incident. I was not particularly pleased that I found out much later, however I was now able to support him emotionally and financially. We stayed by his side while he attended rehab and support groups. The day of his court case was his sister, Sarah's, twentieth birthday, and she never lets him forget it. It's now a joke between them, and I was so relieved that he didn't have to serve time in jail. At least we can all now put the past behind us as Lindsay has bravely turned his life around and is working towards helping others do the same. I believe our love and support helped him to turn his life around.

My mother said to me many years ago that we are there to guide and teach our children until about the age of 16, then after that, we are there to pick up the pieces if need be, and hopefully they've been given all the tools they need to handle life. I would say that I've probably become stronger as a person with all that we've been through as a family. Other people go through worse things, so at the end of the day, we are okay. Lindsay has done a great job getting through this and will be able to help people in the future.

You alone can do it, but you can't do it alone!

I believe we all have the tools to help us navigate our challenges in life. Though sometimes, we need the support and knowledge of others to show us how to tap into our inner strengths and knowing. You are the most important person in your life, and for you to be healthy, you need to put yourself first. Below are suggestions on where to find help if needed, with tools and habits to enhance your life.

Where to find help and support:

Thorne Harbour Health – Support for the LGBTIQ+ community including HIV
Ph: (03) 9865 6700
Website: thorneharbour.org

Lifeline – Crisis support and suicide prevention - available 24/7
Ph: 13 11 14

Beyond Blue – Support for mental health issues
Ph: 1300 22 4636
Website: beyondblue.org.au/getsupport

Go-to person:

Do you have a go-to person/s? This is someone you can turn to in a crisis that you can trust and will be there to support you with no judgement. It can be more than one person. For example, you can nominate someone at work for work issues, and a family member or friend for personal issues. When being challenged, it can sometimes be difficult to make decisions at that time. Now choose your go-to person/s, but let them know they are your chosen person, to avoid any confusion if you need to contact them.

Effective strategies to maintain self-care:

Physical self-care
- Eat healthy and regularly (breakfast, lunch and dinner)
- Exercise
- Meditate
- Get regular medical care for prevention
- Get medical care when needed
- Get massages
- Dance, swim, walk, run, play sports, sing or do some other physical activity that is fun
- Embrace your sexuality – by yourself or with a partner

- Get enough sleep
- Wear clothes that you like and feel good in
- Take vacations, whether longer breaks or mini-vacations and day trips
- Make time away from technology

Psychological self-care

- Make time for self-reflection
- Write in a journal
- Read literature that is unrelated to work
- Do something at which you are not an expert or in charge
- Decrease stress in your life
- Let others know different aspects of you
- Notice your inner voice – listen to your thoughts, judgements, beliefs, attitudes and feelings
- Engage your intelligence in a new area. For example, go to an art museum, history exhibition, sports event, auction or theatre performance
- Practice receiving from others
- Be curious
- Say 'no' to extra responsibilities sometimes

Why and how to meditate:

For thousands of years people have used meditation to move beyond the mind's stress-inducing thoughts and emotional upsets into the peace and clarity of present moment awareness. The variety of meditation techniques, traditions and technologies is almost infinite, but the essence of meditation is singular: the cultivation of mindful awareness and expanded consciousness.

Some benefits of meditation:

Lower stress – There's lots of evidence these days that excess stress causes many illnesses and makes other illnesses worse. Mindfulness decreases stress.

Focus your mind – It can be frustrating to have our mind stray off what we're doing and be pulled in six directions. Meditation hones our innate ability to focus.

Reduce brain chatter – The nattering, chattering voice in our head seems to never leave us alone. Isn't it time we gave it a little break?

Meditation at home is simple, the instructions below will get you started:

- You can access music through Spotify or YouTube for free or you can meditate in silence. Guided meditations are great if your mind wanders too much – *1 Giant Mind app, Headspace app, Guided Mind app* or *Smiling Mind app*. Make sure to put your phone on 'Do Not Disturb' and silence to avoid interruptions.
- Find a room that is quiet. If it's cold you can put a blanket over or around you as it's hard to meditate if you are cold. You may even like to sit outside in nature if it's a nice day.
- Sit on a chair that has a straight back, place your feet flat on the floor (legs uncrossed). Put a pillow under your feet if you can't reach the floor properly.
- You can set a timer or choose a number of meditation tracks to listen to. It's up to you how long you meditate – 5 to 10 minutes or more every day will be advantageous.

- Start the timer and music, close your eyes lightly and place your hands on top of your legs with palms facing up.
- Let go of everyday thoughts (shopping list, today's meeting, what's for dinner). If these types of thoughts come in, acknowledge them then let them pass through. Bring yourself back by listening to the music or concentrating on your breath. You may like to ask a question in your mind and see what comes through, or you just need to relax and revive so slip into the music to give your mind a break.
- At the end of the meditation, close down by surrounding yourself in a protective bubble of white light for a couple of minutes.
- Have a drink of water once you have finished your meditation – this will help ground you.

You are now ready to face a new day!

Remember, do not be hard on yourself if your mind easily wanders as this is normal. Meditation needs to be practiced on a regular basis to get amazing results, but it's definitely worth the effort as excessive stress, depression and anxiety is debilitating.

If you are really time poor and catch public transport, meditation can be done while on the train, bus or tram. You can pop your sunglasses on and no one will know the difference – just be careful not to miss your stop! If you drive to work and can't find an area that is quiet enough for meditation, you can meditate in your car.

The two meditations below will help to get you started.

Centre, Ground and Balance meditation

This meditation is used when you're feeling a bit scattered or lightheaded, as it will help to center, ground and balance your energy.

Sit in the meditation position you prefer, chair or cushion, and start the music. Spend about two minutes on each section.

Centre – Imagine a white light coming in through the top of the head down to the base of the spine, continue the white light through into the ground beneath you.

Ground – Imagine roots growing out of the bottom of your feet to three feet into the ground. You may feel a little bit of tingling in your feet – this is normal as the energy moves through.

Balance – Imagine a triangle that runs under you, up the left-hand side of your body to approx. one foot above your head and down the right-hand side of your body.

Finish off by imagining you are sitting in a rainbow bubble of protection.

Figure 8 meditation (letting go)

Try this meditation when wanting to let go of negative people, thoughts or incidents.

Sit in the meditation position you prefer, in a chair or on a cushion, and start the music.

Begin by breathing white light in through your nose and black out through your mouth for seven breaths.

Next, imagine the figure 8 and place the bottom of the 8 around your chest area with the top of the 8 out in front of you. Place a person, negative thought or incident inside the top circle of the figure 8.

Once this is done, imagine cutting through the middle of the figure 8 with a big pair of scissors or even an axe if you want. Let the top of the figure 8 float off into the darkness as you don't need it anymore in your life.

If you wish, you can have a conversation with the person/s before you cut through the middle of the 8. All you are letting go of is the negative impact someone or something has on your life and you no longer want to waste energy on it. You can still love that person; you're just releasing the negative effects on you.

I want to leave you with these thoughts from Albert Einstein:

1. Stay away from negative people. They have a problem for every solution.

2. We cannot solve our problems with the same thinking we used when we created them.

3. A person who never made a mistake never tried anything new.

4. You never stop failing until you stop trying.

5. Life is like riding a bicycle. To keep your balance, you must keep moving.

6. Two things are infinite: the universe and human stupidity, and I'm not sure about the universe.

7. Insanity is doing the same thing over and over again and expecting different results.

8. Weak people revenge. Strong people forgive. Intelligent people ignore.

9. Logic will get you from A to B. Imagination will take you everywhere.

About the author

Anne Considine has been married to her husband, Paul, for 36 years, and together they have three children, Chris, Anthony and Laura. Both of their boys are gay which inspired Anne to connect with and write other people's stories to bring to light the challenges they have faced and overcome. Anne's work as a Spiritual Counsellor through her business, Purple Haven, has helped her relate to the men who have entrusted her with their stories. She felt their voices needed to be heard and understood in the hope that it may alleviate someone's pain in the future, whether it be someone struggling with their sexuality or a parent of someone gay that wants to garner more insight into the mind of their son, brother, father or friend.

Anne has also worked in Homecare at Thorne Harbour Health (previously known as the Victorian Aids Council) and is now a volunteer. She is a strong supporter of the LGBTIQ community, and longs for the day that we can love whoever we want to love with no judgement!

Acknowledgements

Writing this book has been a wild ride of ups and downs! Throw COVID-19 into the mix and it's a crazy combo. I could not have achieved this book if it wasn't for the brave and beautiful men who were willing to tell me their stories and giving us an insight into a world that most of us can only imagine. There were times where I was brought to tears and times that we laughed out loud as we worked together. I thank you all for your honesty and trusting me with your stories. I also hope that you received some healing by opening up your hearts to me. You truly are inspiring to all.

To my husband, Paul, I want to thank you for believing in me and supporting me through the times when I doubted myself. You've always been my champion and for that I'm forever grateful. Chris, Anthony and Laura, thanks for being the best human beings I know. You challenge me, but you make me laugh at the same time. Your openness and honesty are your best attributes and I'd be lost without you.

For those of you who have assisted in the editing process before the book actually got to the Editor, a big thank you! Sue Dyson and Margaret Burn, I appreciate your patience, attention to detail and constructive comments. I'm sure your diligence has made the Editor's job much easier.

To my talented nephew, James Rendall, who drew the beautiful artwork on the front cover of the book, I feel privileged that you allowed me to use your work.

This is a big thank you to my friends who have listened to me talk about the stories and any issues I have come across while writing. Kathleen Pennicard, Livia Vidotto, Carmel Crossley and Mary Amerena, your unconditional friendship and kindness have always been highly valued by me. Even after all these years when I come up with a new idea or thought, you still listen intently and without judgement. I'm so fortunate to have you all in my life!

To my personal trainer, Tiffany Christie, who kept me in shape both physically and emotionally while writing this book. She motivated me by factoring in writing time as part of my training schedule; to keep me going when it was the last thing I wanted to do.

To the staff at Little Sister Café on Bay Street, Brighton – in particular, Sawan, the owner, and Alisha, the best barista ever, our brainstorming and your infectious enthusiasm spurred me on to complete this book. A big thank you to you all, as you got me through the writing process with amazing support – and coffee.

Last but not least, I appreciate the encouragement, guidance and patience from Natasa Denman and her team at Ultimate 48

Acknowledgements

Hour Author. If it wasn't for their hard work, expertise in self publishing and holding me accountable, I doubt I would have finished this book at all.

Call to action

It's time let go of the past and embrace the future, as life is too short to be constantly unhappy or stressed!

Relax, breathe and tell me all about it

If you or, someone you know, may be struggling with life, then book in to see me at Purple Haven in Melbourne, Australia, where you can unload (or dump, if preferable) your burdens in a safe, caring, non-judgemental and relaxed environment. If you feel confused, overwhelmed, anxious, depressed, angry or just plain unhappy, let's begin to shed some light on the core of the problem. Other areas of life to uncover could be identifying negative patterns of behaviour, finding your voice or passion. They say a problem shared, is a problem halved – that's always a good start. The scope of modalities used are: Discussion, Reiki, Meditation, Oracle Card Readings and Flower Essences.

To book in for a one-on-one session or for further details, please go to my website: www.purplehaven.com.au . You will also find options to purchase more copies of *From Outside the Closet*.

If you would like me to speak about this book or my work, I am available for speaking engagements or interviews – contact details on my website or email me at: purplehaven9@gmail.com

Testimonials

I'm thrilled that my dear friend, Anne Considine, has written her first book, and has been able to share not only her story, but other people's journey as well. Over the many years I have known her, she has always been there to listen and guide me, but most of all, has helped me navigate through challenges that life often throws in one's way. As she has helped me in the past, I know there are many more people out there who could use Anne's guidance to help them through their own journey of life.

Livia Vidotto AMC

What a beautiful soul Anne is, and what a powerful gift she has! Anne's expertise and guidance helped me overcome a challenging hurdle in my life. I am so grateful that our paths aligned.

Mimi Giordano